D0115708

"Expert bariatric surgeon Flancbaum h[...] reassuring guide for those considering the surgery. He clearly outlines the surgical options, explaining each type along with its risks and possible complications, as well as expected outcomes. He also explains what to expect before, during, and after surgery, discussing selection of a surgeon, insurance coverage, the surgery itself, pain control, diet, and (rarely) reoperation. Resources and recipes are appended."

—*Library Journal*

"This book is a must-read for anyone considering weight loss surgery or just exploring treatment options for morbid obesity. It's well-researched, authoritative and easy-to-read. The authors include one of the top WLS surgeons and a writer who had weight loss surgery, so they know what they're talking about. Every question a reader might have is anticipated, and ably answered. A great resource!"

—Belinda Hulin, features editor, *Florida Times-Union*

"Finally, an authoritative, comprehensive guide from a real expert. The insurance chapter alone is worth the asking price."

—Barbara Stras, Coordinator, Kansas City
Weight Loss Surgery Support Group

THE DOCTOR'S GUIDE TO WEIGHT LOSS SURGERY
A Bantam Book

PUBLISHING HISTORY
Fredonia Press trade paperback edition / June 2001
Bantam trade paperback edition / September 2003

Published by Bantam Dell a division of
Random House, Inc.
New York, New York

Book design by Joseph Rutt
Cover design by Beverly Leung
Interior illustrations by Virginia Cantarella

Library of Congress Cataloging-in-Publication Data
Flancbaum, Louis J.
    The doctor's guide to weight loss surgery : how to make the
decision that could save your life / Louis J. Flancbaum and
Erica Manfred with Deborah Flancbaum.
        p. cm.
    Included bibliographical references and index.
    ISBN 0-553-38246-2
    1. Obesity—Surgery—Popular works.   2. Gastrointestinal
system—Surgery—Popular works.   I. Manfred, Erica.
II. Flancbaum, Deborah.   III. Title.

RD540.F63 2003
617.4'3—dc21   2003051892

Manufactured in the United States of America
Published simultaneously in Canada

RRH   10 9 8 7 6 5 4 3 2 1

THE
DOCTOR'S
GUIDE
TO
WEIGHT LOSS
SURGERY

How to Make the Decision That Could Save Your Life

Louis Flancbaum, M.D.
and Erica Manfred with Deborah Flancbaum

BANTAM BOOKS
NEW YORK TORONTO LONDON SYDNEY AUCKLAND

To all of my patients who have entrusted their lives to me and who, in addition to teaching me much of what I know about bariatric surgery, have taught me a much more important lesson about life. By observing and getting to know them, I have witnessed what it is like to suffer from a chronic illness such as severe obesity and how to be courageous, persevere, and eventually flourish in the face of adversity.

Louis Flancbaum, M.D.

The information in this book about the risks and rewards of weight loss surgery for the morbidly obese is based on an in-depth review of the current scientific literature, interviews with experts, and the experience of the authors. The authors have written this book because they believe that the more fully informed persons are about weight loss surgery, the better they will be able to make an informed choice.

They have worked to ensure that all information in the book concerning types of procedures, surgical complications, effect on co-morbid conditions, nutritional guidelines, etc., is accurate as of the time of publication.

The book is intended only as a resource guide to help you make informed decisions; it is not meant to replace the advice of a physician. Always seek competent medical help for any health condition or if you have any questions about a specific procedure or health recommendation. Be aware that as medical research and practice advance, therapeutic approaches may change or evolve. This is why a physician is the only reliable source of such advice.

ACKNOWLEDGMENTS

This book owes a lot to the many, many people who pitched in to help get it into print. Most volunteered their time and expertise as a favor, which was amazing, gratifying, and wonderful. We are incredibly grateful to . . .

Barb Stras, leader of the Kansas City weight loss surgery support group and a marketing expert, who gave unstintingly of her time and great advice. She was always there with encouragement and support when the going got rough.

Virginia Cantarella, one of the best medical illustrators in the business, who contributed the amazing medical illustrations gratis. When we asked how much she would charge, she said, "You couldn't afford me, so I'll do them for free." We believe her illustrations are the best ever done of the various weight loss surgeries.

Mitch Sewall, cook extraordinaire, who devoted an enormous amount of time and energy to learning about weight loss surgery in order to come up with recipes that would work for postop patients. We truly appreciate his tasty recipes, which will give people who read the book hope that eating after weight loss surgery doesn't have to be dull but can be a gourmet experience.

Toni Colarusso, nutritionist at St. Luke's–Roosevelt Hospital, who spent many long hours analyzing the nutritional values of the recipes.

Nicolle Siegel, nutritionist for gastric bypass and duodenal switch patients in Mt. Sinai Hospital, New York, who offered her extensive expertise on post-op nutrition. She gave us advice about such important issues as the post-op diet for duodenal-switch patients, heading off nutritional deficiencies, and how to deal with them if they occur.

Tony C. Merry, a lawyer with Palmer Volkema Thomas in Columbus, Ohio, who was extremely helpful when it came to sorting out the intricacies of the law regarding health-insurance coverage for weight loss surgery.

Finally, Leslie Rutledge and Linda Saxe-Turner, who shared their expertise in dealing with HMOs.

CONTENTS

This is a particularly good time for a book aimed at those who may be considering weight loss surgery. We now understand that obesity is a chronic disease caused by many different factors. Scientists have discovered numerous genes that contribute to weight gain, and, at last count, over 200 genes and gene markers have been identified. There clearly are biochemical differences in the bodies of people with obesity compared to nonobese people.

If an obese person loses weight by standard medical therapy, his or her biochemistry does not return to that of a nonobese person. In fact, biochemical changes occur that tend to favor weight gain and fat gain. Although the genetic contribution to obesity is clearly important, it probably causes only about 40 percent of the obesity in the total population. The other 60 percent may be attributed to environmental causes. The presence of an abundance of inexpensive, good tasting, high calorie, high fat, rapidly available food allows the genetic traits present in most of us to come through as an increase in body weight. More ominous, recent research demonstrates that certain viruses produce obesity in animals and there are links for at least some of these viruses to human obesity.

It is not surprising that the incidence of obesity in the United States and across the world is exploding. In the last twenty years the percentage of adult Americans with medically significant obesity has increased by 75 percent, and more than 55 percent of Americans are overweight. The World Health Organization has declared that there is a *global epidemic* of obesity. The number of people who meet the criteria for weight loss surgery is now almost 5 percent of the population. Nevertheless, there is still great fear and misunderstanding about weight loss surgery. Many patients in my practice refuse even to discuss the option. Many physicians will not consider sending their patients for this surgery. These attitudes are based on the belief that none of the treatments for obesity is effective and that any treatment for obesity other than diet and exercise may be dangerous.

The reality is that there has been a great deal of research on treatment for obesity, and we now understand that weight loss surgery is the single most effective treatment for individuals who have the severest form of the disease of obesity. Long-term studies on patients who have undergone weight loss surgery show that extensive weight loss may be attained by the majority of patients. Complications of obesity, such as diabetes, high blood pressure, sleep apnea, arthritis, and gastroesophageal reflux disease (heartburn) improve markedly or disappear. One study even shows that weight loss surgery decreases the higher death rate associated with obesity.

The Doctor's Guide to Weight Loss Surgery: How to Make the Decision That Could Save Your Life explains how the severity of obesity is graded and who is a candidate for weight loss surgery. In practical terms, it describes the types of operations used for obesity and the advantages and disadvantages of each. Each operation has a balance of benefits and risks that should be understood by anyone considering weight loss surgery. Patients need long-term follow-up after surgery, because some of the complications may not show up immediately.

The book takes the prospective patient through the whole process of weight loss surgery, from the pre-surgical evaluation, to what will occur in the hospital at each step along the way, how long the hospitalization will be, how long before normal activities may be resumed, and what to watch out for in the months and years after surgery. Eating after surgery may need to be different than before, so guidelines are given. Finally, practical advice is given on choosing a surgeon and a follow-up program, as well as steps that can be taken to improve the chances that the insurance company or third-party payer will pay for the surgery.

In summary, this book takes the mystery out of weight loss surgery and allows patients to make an informed decision about this important step in the treatment of their disease. It is a much-needed guide to the most effective treatment for extreme obesity and should be read by all severely overweight people who are considering surgery as a treatment option.

Richard L. Atkinson, M.D.
President
American Obesity Association
April 2001

THE
DOCTOR'S
GUIDE
TO
WEIGHT LOSS
SURGERY

I used to think that weight loss surgery (WLS) was the last resort for desperate, self-destructive, fat people with no self-control and little self-esteem. I'd heard about all the deaths that resulted from the original intestinal-bypass procedure thirty years ago and was convinced that this type of surgery was perpetrated by irresponsible "quacks" on vulnerable, unsuspecting patients. Accepting my weight, I vowed to persevere and be successful despite it. However, I was distraught about my health. My ever-increasing weight was causing worsening diabetes, higher cholesterol, painful arthritis, and intolerable heartburn. I knew I had to do something to control my weight, but what? I'd tried every commercial and fad diet known to humankind, shed hundreds of pounds, and regained even more.

Then I discovered that an old friend had successfully undergone WLS, lost over one hundred pounds, and was now thin and healthy. When I first heard about his surgery I was horrified, assuming he'd ruined his life for the brass ring of thinness. But, after seeing him doing so well, I began having second thoughts. Each visit to the endocrinologist was accompanied by higher blood-sugar readings, meaning that I was closer to needing insulin injections. I fantasized about having the surgery. Then my dentist had WLS and the pounds kept dropping off her. As she became thinner, her personality changed. Where she had always been remote and aloof, she suddenly became bubbly, happy, and talkative. As she was filling a cavity during one visit, she told me that the surgery had changed her life and she was sorry she hadn't done it years earlier. I was stunned that a physical procedure could have such a profound psychological effect, even before she reached her goal weight.

I called my friend and we spoke for a long time. A lawyer and extremely thorough investigator, he had researched WLS exhaustively and learned that it was safe and effective as long as you chose a qualified surgeon and were vigilant about taking your vitamins. I'd been taking daily doses of pills for years, so that was not going to deter me.

I couldn't argue with his or my dentist's results. I became very excited about the prospect of having surgery. Perhaps having WLS really was a way to reverse the terrible downhill slide my health was taking.

Even after talking at length to my friend and my dentist, I still kept waffling for over a year. I was scared of being cut open, of anesthesia, and especially of pain. I scheduled surgery three times with three different surgeons before I finally took the plunge. One factor that helped me reach my decision was reading the OSSG@egroups.com (Obesity Surgery Support Group) list on the Internet day after day, month after month, and seeing how many people just like me—many in much worse health than me—had undergone WLS, lived through it, and were extremely happy they'd done it. Finally, I realized if they could do it, so could I.

I had gastric bypass surgery in January 1999 and have lost 70 pounds, about 60 percent of my excess weight. Although I'm still overweight, I can do everything I want to do, including run up and down stairs, bend over, get up off the floor, walk for two miles without getting winded, and, most important, keep up with my five-year-old. My quality of life has been transformed. The best news, however, is that my blood sugar is finally under control with just a small amount of medication.

Once my choice was made, I wanted to learn as much as I could about WLS. I searched the Internet, went to libraries, read medical literature and lay publications. Over and over, I hit dead ends. There was little high-quality information for the layperson about WLS that described the different operations, their pros and cons and long-term effects. Nothing was available offering advice about selecting a competent surgeon, a comprehensive program, or dealing with insurance carriers—often the major obstacles to overcome prior to WLS. This book was written as a result of my experience, to provide a useful resource and fill a void for others contemplating WLS. My collaborator is Dr. Louis Flancbaum, a general surgeon and nationally recognized authority in bariatric surgery. He is Chief of the Division of Bariatric Surgery at St. Luke's–Roosevelt Hospital Center in New York City and associate professor of clinical surgery at the College of Physicians and Surgeons of Columbia University. Dr. Flancbaum, who has performed over 1,200 bariatric surgical procedures in his twelve years in the field, has made many national and international presentations and has published over one hundred scientific journal articles and book chapters. His study, with Dr. Patricia Choban, of patient satisfaction after weight loss surgery received national attention.

Dr. Flancbaum's skills as a surgeon are formidable. He performs the gastric bypass in an amazing forty-five minutes to an hour, without sacrificing technique—making it a safer operation. But he is more than just an expert surgeon—he has demonstrated a devotion to the problems of obese people. As he expressed to me, "Society doesn't value morbidly obese people. They're considered almost subhuman in today's culture. When I see what my patients go through I feel a strong sense of empathy for them."

Unlike most surgeons, who have little contact with their patients after they leave the operating room, Dr. Flancbaum enjoys getting to know and work with his patients over the long term. Weight loss surgery, unlike most, isn't just a one-shot deal but takes a long-term commitment by the surgeon and his staff to succeed. Also, unlike other surgical specialties in which the surgeon doesn't get to see the effects of his work, Dr. Flancbaum gets tremendous satisfaction from witnessing the total transformation he makes in the lives of his patients. His extensive knowledge of both gastric bypass surgery and the disease of obesity made him the perfect expert to collaborate with. He also has a gift for explaining complicated medical jargon in simple language the layperson can understand, as you will see throughout this book.

The Doctor's Guide to Weight Loss Surgery: How to Make the Decision That Could Save Your Life is a comprehensive reference for those considering WLS. We have provided detailed information about the health risks associated with severe obesity and its treatments. The various WLS procedures are described, along with their anticipated outcomes, risks, benefits, and complications. Additional chapters offer tips to help guide prospective surgical candidates through the process of selecting a bariatric surgeon and weight loss program and obtaining insurance approval.

Finally, a number of personal vignettes from Dr. Flancbaum's practice have been included to provide a human connection and "moral support." All the stories are true, but the names and other identifying information have been changed to protect the privacy of the patients, except for my real-life story and the story of Denise Rasley, which comprises the penultimate chapter. The sentiments expressed are representative of what is repeatedly heard from WLS patients, in support groups and elsewhere.

It is our hope that this book will allow people suffering with clinically severe obesity to make an informed decision about WLS, which can dramatically improve their health and well-being.

Erica Manfred

Note on Style
When the first person is used in the body of this book, it is Dr. Flancbaum speaking about his own surgical practice. Other first-person experiences will be differentiated by italics or introduced separately.

OBESITY: AMERICA'S DISEASE

I've been fat since I was a baby. My entire family is fat. Who knows if it's our genes or our eating habits or a combination of both. I just know that being fat is a horrible way to have to live.

Sara P., 43, 360 lbs. pre-op; 200 lbs. 2 years post-op

When I walk around at the mall with my kids, I have to admit that I look at people who are obese. It reminds me of how I looked and felt before the operation. It's amazing how many people there are out there suffering from this when there is something that can be done about it.

Tim W., 50, 400 lbs. pre-op; 230 lbs. 18 months post-op

> *Disease (noun)—a specific illness or disorder characterized by a recognizable set of signs and symptoms, attributable to heredity, infection, diet, or environment.* (Mosby's Medical, Nursing, and Allied Health Dictionary, Fifth Edition)

Contrary to popular opinion, obesity is *not* a personality disorder resulting from a lack of individual willpower or self-control. Rather, it is a chronic disease characterized by the accumulation of excess body fat, which can be detrimental to health. Obesity is distinguished from *overweight*, which does not take body composition into consideration. Many athletes are overweight, but because their excess weight is predominantly comprised of muscle, not fat tissue, they are not obese.

SOME FACTS ABOUT OBESITY

The worldwide incidence of obesity is increasing. In 1998, the World Health Organization published *Obesity: Preventing and Managing the Global Epidemic,* which classified obesity as a growing epidemic. In the United States, obesity is the most common chronic disease, affecting one-third of all Americans, including children, and its prevalence has been steadily increasing for the past twenty years. In Europe, Australia, New Zealand, the Middle East, and the remaining portions of the Americas, the occurrence of obesity appears to be increasing and is now between 10 and 20 percent. The prevalence of obesity is still fairly low in China, Japan, and many countries in Africa.

During the 1970s, the National Center for Health Statistics found that approximately 45 percent of all adult Americans were overweight and 14 percent were obese. These figures stayed relatively constant for over a decade. Armed with this information at the beginning of the 1990s, the Department of Health and Human Resources published *Healthy People 2000,* a policy statement outlining our national public-health priorities and goals as we entered the new millennium. The initiatives recommended included: reducing the incidence of overweight and obesity by 20 percent; improving the diagnosis and treatment of several obesity-related conditions, such as diabetes, coronary artery disease (hardening of the arteries), hypertension (high blood pressure), and hyperlipidemia (elevated serum cholesterol and blood lipids); and increasing the amount of regular aerobic exercise engaged in by adults and children.

When the National Center for Health Statistics repeated its survey in the mid-1990s, it found that the prevalence of overweight had increased from 47 percent to 54 percent (57 million people), with the prevalence of obesity increasing from 15 to 22 percent (40 million people). Moreover, the prevalence of severe obesity rose from 4.5 percent to 8 percent of the population (Table 1-1). In 1995, the Institute of Medicine, in its publication

Weighing the Options, referred to obesity as an *epidemic*. It is currently estimated that there are approximately 127 million overweight or obese adults in the United States. Of these, 30 million are obese with a Body Mass Index of 30 to 34, 23 million are severely obese, with a Body Mass Index of 35 to 39, and 10 million suffer from morbid or clinically severe obesity, with a Body Mass Index above 40. (We will discuss the Body Mass Index, or BMI, in Chapter 2.)

Among American youth, the prevalence of obesity has skyrocketed during the past two decades, from just under 4 percent in children (six to eleven years) and 6 percent in teenagers (twelve to nineteen years) to 15 percent in children and 15 percent in adolescents. The prevalence of overweight is also extremely high among youth, being 40 percent in Native Americans, 30 percent in African Americans and Hispanics, 25 percent in whites, and 20 percent in Asian-Americans. As with adults, obesity in youth is associated with a number of medical problems, including type II diabetes, hypertension, asthma, sleep apnea, orthopedic problems, psychological problems, and negative social stigmata.

The exact cause of obesity remains unknown, but multiple factors, genetic and environmental, appear to contribute. Afflicting individuals of all ages, genders, races, and ethnic groups, obesity is associated with numerous medical problems and can have a relatively benign or malignant course. Obesity increases steadily with age in both men and women, and it is more common in women than men. It affects African-American and Mexican-American women more than Caucasians or Asian-Americans. A strong genetic linkage exists among the Pima Indians, who live in the Southwestern United States.

Children born to obese parents are more likely to become obese than children born to thin parents. Studies of adopted children have shown that their tendency toward obesity is more related to the weight of their birth parents than their adoptive parents. Furthermore, in studies of twins who were raised separately, the ultimate weight of each sibling tended to be more similar to each other than to that of their nonbiological, adopted family members. Nevertheless, it is likely that these genetic factors merely predispose individuals to obesity but do not guarantee its development. The disease becomes manifest only in the presence of the proper environmental triggers, which are related to several factors, including culture, diet, and physical activity.

Over the past few centuries, Western industrialized societies have placed a progressively greater value on thinness. Television and magazine advertisements equate beauty with thinness. By contrast, the robust bodies of the women glorified in masterpieces throughout the Middle Ages and Renaissance would be considered obese by our standards. On the other hand, in poorer, underdeveloped cultures, where famine is common, obesity is perceived as a sign of wealth and is therefore associated with greater sexual attractiveness.

Diet and exercise also affect the onset and development of obesity. High-fat diets, which are prevalent in wealthier, Western cultures, increase the prevalence of obesity. Modernization of society and the development of ever more advanced technology have led to a progressive decrease in physical activity. Inventions such as the automobile, elevator, escalator, remote control, and wireless communication all decrease the amount of physical activity we perform daily. Similarly, children reared on television, video games, and computers are more likely to become obese than those who exercise regularly.

Table 1-1: Increase in the Prevalence of Overweight and Obesity in the United States

Weight Category*	1976–1980	1988–1994	1999–2000	Number Americans
Overweight	32 percent	32 percent	34 percent	64 million
Obese	10 percent	14 percent	16 percent	30 million
Severely Obese	3 percent	5 percent	9 percent	23 million
Morbid Obesity	2 percent	3 percent	5 percent	10 million
Total Population	47 percent	54 percent	64 percent	127 million

* Classification based upon World Health Organization
American Obesity Association: www.aoa.org/subs/fastfacts/obesity_US.shtml

THE HIGH COST OF OBESITY

The economic cost of obesity is enormous. An estimated $70 billion is spent annually in the United States on the treatment of obesity and its related conditions. This sum represents about 8 percent of the total health-care budget, or one out of every twelve dollars spent on health care. In addition, another $33 billion is expended on commercial weight loss programs each year, despite the fact that there is no available evidence suggesting that they are effective in producing long-term weight loss. Annually, the cost of obesity treatment exceeds $100 billion. At any given time, an estimated 40 percent of women and 25 percent of men are trying to lose weight, with an additional 30 percent involved in weight maintenance.

The significance of obesity as a public-health problem is related to its association with a number of complicating (or co-morbid) medical conditions. Obesity alone is a risk factor for premature death, with risk increasing in direct proportion to weight. Furthermore, obesity is causally related to diabetes, hypertension, coronary artery disease, stroke, sleep apnea, venous disease, gallstones, gastroesophageal reflux (heartburn), osteoarthritis, urinary stress incontinence, menstrual irregularity, infertility, depression, and several types of cancer. Many of these health problems improve or completely resolve with weight loss. Ironically, many insurance carriers and the federal government continue to refuse to pay for obesity treatments (diets, drugs, behavior modification, and surgery) but willingly expend funds to treat diseases that result from obesity.

Obesity takes a social and psychological toll on its victims. Obese individuals face discrimination in school, the workplace, the media, and in the health-care system. Many health-insurance plans do not cover obesity treatment or, if they do, the benefits are severely reduced or restricted. The decisions of insurance and managed-care companies in this regard are often arbitrary and ignore established medical evidence. No other group of individuals is stigmatized to the same degree as the obese and forced to jump through so many hoops in order to receive authorization for the care of a chronic debilitating disease. Morbidly obese people seeking weight loss surgery have to document every diet they have ever been on in addition to undergoing psychological screening to make sure they will comply with the dietary requirements after surgery. Smokers suffering from coronary artery disease in need of open-heart surgery do not need to present letters from their physicians verifying that they have stopped smoking nor do they need to undergo psychological screening to ensure that they will modify their diet and engage in a cardiac rehabilitation program after surgery. Physicians and other health-care practitioners involved in the treatment of obesity are also stigmatized, still often referred to as "quacks."

Recently, inroads have been made into the causes and treatment of obesity. Identification of several genes and their corresponding hormones, such as leptin, that are in part responsible for obesity have confirmed that it has a biological basis, helping to reduce the misconception that obesity is a behavioral or psychological disorder. Several promising new drugs and drug classes have been introduced to treat obesity. However, these medications face severe hurdles before they can become available to the general public. They have strict restrictions against long-term use, often based on misconceptions rather than scientific evidence that they are addictive. Safe and effective surgical techniques have been devised that produce long-term weight control for the most severely obese individuals and result in significant improvements in associated medical problems. The beneficial effects of surgery in severe obesity have been evaluated, confirmed, and endorsed by the National Institutes of Health, the World Health Organization, the American Obesity Association, and Shape Up America! Nevertheless, much still remains to be done to improve the treatment of obesity and access to treatment.

2

ARE YOU OBESE?

The first time I saw the word obese *used to describe me was when I sneaked a look at my medical chart when my doctor walked out of the room. I was shocked. I knew I was fat—but it was hard to accept the fact that I was that far gone.*

Maggie L., 54, 384 lbs. pre-op; 265 lbs. 3 years post-op

I never saw the term morbidly obese *until I read it in a magazine. It didn't take me long to understand what it meant. If I didn't begin to take care of my health—I was not going to live to a ripe old age.*

Karen K., 38, 288 lbs. pre-op; 179 lbs. 1 year post-op

The medical, psychological, social, and economic consequences of obesity are directly related to body size. The greater the degree of obesity, the greater the health risk. In order to more accurately predict the increased health risk associated with obesity, it is necessary to accurately describe the degree of obesity.

BODY MASS INDEX, OR BMI

Obesity can be defined in several ways. In the past, people referred to height–weight tables (such as those published by the Metropolitan Life Insurance Company) to determine if their weight was appropriate for their height. The weights were often corrected for "frame size" (small, medium, large). In recent years, height–weight tables have fallen out of favor within the medical and scientific communities and have been replaced by a method that more accurately accounts for the relative contributions of height and weight—called the Body Mass Index, or BMI. (BMI is generally expressed as kg/m², but for the sake of simplicity we will omit the kg/m² notation in the remainder of the book.)

To calculate your BMI:

Multiply your weight in pounds by 705.
Divide that number by your height in inches.
Divide that number by your height in inches again.

You can also calculate your BMI by using the accompanying Table 2-1.

IDEAL AND EXCESS BODY WEIGHT

Although BMI is the preferred method for describing one's health risk as it relates to weight, the concepts of Ideal (or Desirable) Body Weight (IBW) and Excess Body Weight (EBW) are simple ones. The notion of an IBW, which is the ideal amount that a person should weigh, arose from the use of height–weight tables. Several formulas to estimate IBW exist, but the simplest is:

IBW (Women) = 100 lbs. for the first 5 ft. of height, + or − 5 lbs. for each inch above or below. (For example, a woman 5 ft. 2 in. tall has an IBW = 110 lbs.)

IBW (Men) = 106 lbs. for the first 5 ft. of height, + or − 6 lbs. for each inch above or below. (For example, a man 5 ft. 2 in. tall has an IBW = 118 lbs.)

EBW, which is the amount that one is overweight, is calculated as follows:

EBW = Actual body weight (ABW) minus IBW

In addition to estimating how much a person "should weigh" and how much he or she is overweight, IBW and EBW are most useful in estimating how much weight an individual can reasonably expect to lose following WLS. You can reasonably expect to lose at least 50 percent of your EBW following WLS.

ASSESSING THE RELATIONSHIP BETWEEN WEIGHT AND HEALTH RISK

A normal BMI is between 19 and 25, and beyond this level, health risks increase steadily. In 1998, the World Health

Table 2-1: BMI Table

	Height (inches)																				
Wt.	60	61	62	63	64	65	66	67	68	69	70	71	72	73	74	75	76	77	78	79	80
140	27	26	26	25	24	23	22	22	21	21	20										
150	29	28	27	26	26	25	24	23	23	22	21	21	20	20							
160	31	30	29	28	27	26	26	25	24	23	23	22	22	21	20	20					
170	33	32	31	30	29	28	27	26	26	25	24	24	23	22	22	21	21	20			
180	35	34	33	32	31	30	29	28	27	26	26	25	24	24	23	22	22	21	21	20	20
190	37	36	34	33	32	31	30	29	29	28	27	26	26	25	24	24	23	22	22	21	21
200	39	38	36	35	34	33	32	31	30	29	28	28	27	26	25	25	24	23	23	22	22
210	41	39	38	37	36	35	34	33	32	31	30	29	28	27	27	26	25	25	24	23	23
220	43	41	40	39	38	36	35	34	33	32	31	30	30	29	28	27	27	26	25	25	24
230	45	43	42	40	39	38	37	36	35	34	33	32	31	30	29	29	28	27	26	26	25
240	47	45	44	42	41	40	38	37	36	35	34	33	32	31	31	30	29	28	27	27	26
250	48	47	45	44	43	41	40	39	38	37	36	35	34	33	32	31	30	29	29	28	27
260	50	49	47	46	44	43	42	40	39	38	37	36	35	34	33	32	31	31	30	29	28
270	52	51	49	47	46	45	43	42	41	40	38	37	36	35	34	33	33	32	31	30	29
280	54	53	51	49	48	46	45	43	42	41	40	39	38	37	36	35	34	33	32	31	31
290	56	54	53	51	49	48	46	45	44	43	41	40	39	38	37	36	35	34	33	32	32
300	58	56	54	53	51	49	48	47	45	44	43	42	40	39	38	37	36	35	34	33	33
310	60	58	56	54	53	51	50	48	47	45	44	43	42	41	40	38	37	36	35	35	34
320	62	60	58	56	55	53	51	50	48	47	46	44	43	42	41	40	39	38	37	36	35
330	64	62	60	58	56	54	53	51	50	48	47	46	44	43	42	41	40	39	38	37	36
340	66	64	62	60	58	56	54	53	51	50	48	47	46	44	43	42	41	40	39	38	37
350	68	66	64	62	60	58	56	54	53	51	50	48	47	46	45	43	42	41	40	39	38

Continues on next page

Table 2-1 (Continued)

Height (inches)

Wt.	60	61	62	63	64	65	66	67	68	69	70	71	72	73	74	75	76	77	78	79	80
360	70	68	65	63	61	59	58	56	54	53	51	50	49	47	46	45	43	42	41	40	39
370	72	69	67	65	63	61	59	57	56	54	53	51	50	48	47	46	45	43	42	41	40
380	74	71	69	67	65	63	61	59	57	56	54	53	51	50	48	47	46	45	44	42	41
390	76	73	71	69	66	64	62	61	59	57	56	54	53	51	50	48	47	46	45	44	42
400	78	75	73	70	68	66	64	62	60	59	57	55	54	52	51	50	48	47	46	45	44
410	80	77	74	72	70	68	66	64	62	60	58	57	55	54	52	51	49	48	47	46	45
420	81	79	76	74	72	69	67	65	63	62	60	58	57	55	54	52	51	49	48	47	46
430	83	81	78	76	73	71	69	67	65	63	61	60	58	56	55	53	52	51	49	48	47
440	85	83	80	77	75	73	70	68	66	64	63	61	59	58	56	55	53	52	50	49	48
450	88	84	82	79	77	74	72	70	68	66	64	62	61	59	57	56	54	53	52	50	49
460	90	90	83	81	78	76	74	71	69	67	66	64	62	60	59	57	56	54	53	51	50
470	92	90	85	83	80	77	75	73	71	69	67	65	63	61	60	58	57	55	54	52	51
480	94	91	88	84	82	79	77	74	72	70	68	66	65	63	61	60	58	56	55	54	52
490	96	93	90	87	84	81	78	76	74	72	70	68	66	64	62	61	59	58	56	55	53
500	98	95	92	89	85	82	80	78	76	73	71	69	67	65	64	62	60	59	57	56	54

Organization, in its report *Obesity: Preventing and Managing the Global Epidemic,* proposed a new classification for health risk related to BMI. Individuals with BMIs between 20 and 25 are considered normal. Those with BMIs between 25 and 30 are classified as overweight, with only a mild to moderate increase in health risk. The risk increases as the BMI rises above 30 (obese), 35 (severe obesity), and 40 (morbid or clinically severe obesity). Individuals with a BMI greater than 50 are often referred to as *super obese* and carry the greatest threat to health. There is also a health risk associated with being too thin, with a BMI less than 19. (See Table 2-2.)

People with morbid or clinically severe obesity are at greatest risk for the various associated health problems. In the past, these labels were used when someone was 100 pounds above ideal body weight or twice his or her ideal weight. With more widespread use of BMI to describe health risk, this corresponds to a BMI greater

Table 2-2: Health Risk in Relation to BMI*

BMI (kg/m²)	Obesity Category	Health Risk without Medical Problems	Health Risk with Medical Problems
Below 19	Underweight	Slight	Minimal
19–24	Normal	None	Minimal
25–29	Overweight	Minimal	Moderate
30–34	Obese	Moderate	High
35–39	Severely obese	High	Very High
40–49	Morbidly obese	Very high	Extreme
50+	Super obese	Extreme	Very extreme

* Classification based upon World Health Organization

than 40 or greater than 35 in the presence of life-threatening complications. In general, co-morbid medical conditions are most common in patients with severe and clinically severe/morbid obesity.

When describing the effects of obesity treatment, it is necessary to evaluate weight loss and its impact on associated health risks. A better and more scientifically accurate approach would probably be to estimate how many BMI units one would have to lose in order to lower overall health risk and reach a "healthier weight." However, it is much more understandable to express weight loss in pounds ("I lost 100 pounds") than in BMI units ("My BMI went from 50 to 27").

The various formulas describing weight discussed so far are summarized in Table 2-3.

Table 2-3: Useful Formulas in Weight Loss Surgery

Body Mass Index (BMI) = Weight (kgs) ÷ Height (meters)²; or Weight (pounds) × 705 ÷ Height (inches)²

Ideal Body Weight (IBW)

Women = 100 lbs. for the first 5 ft. of height, + or – 5 lbs. for each inch above or below.

Men = 106 lbs. for the first 5 ft. of height, + or – 6 lbs. for each inch above or below.

Excess body weight (EBW) = Actual body weight (ABW) – IBW

3

WHY OBESITY IS A KILLER DISEASE

I knew that obesity was killing me. My blood pressure was skyrocketing and my diabetes was out of control. I realized that if I didn't get a handle on this thing—my life would soon be over.

Steve P., 54, 337 lbs. pre-op; 214 lbs. 5 years post-op

I felt as if I was eating myself into an early grave. I worked in a senior-citizen center and kept looking around for obese people in their eighties. I couldn't find any—because they were already dead.

Kerry R., 44, 422 lbs. pre-op; 288 lbs. 2½ years post-op

My blood pressure was so high that I was afraid I would have a stroke like my mother. All I wanted to do was live to see my kids grow up.

Larry J., 42, 379 lbs. pre-op; 272 lbs. 1 year post-op

Obesity is an independent risk factor for premature death, with the threat rising as the BMI increases. People with a BMI of 30 have a risk of dying early that is 1.3 times greater than normal-weight individuals. This risk increases to 1.8 times at a BMI of 35, 2.5 times at a BMI of 40, and continues to rise rapidly above that level. When adjusted for age, the increased risk of sudden death appears even more dramatic. In morbidly obese men between 25 and 34 years of age, the risk of premature death is increased twelvefold, sixfold in the 35 to 44 age group, threefold from 45 to 54, and double above 55. It is estimated that obesity and its associated health problems contribute to 300,000 deaths annually in the United States, second only to tobacco and smoking as a causative factor for premature death.

Aside from premature death, obesity is found in conjunction with a variety of associated or co-morbid medical conditions. Several of these conditions can be life-threatening, while others interfere with quality of life.

Several of the potentially life-threatening complications connected with obesity are affected by body shape and fat distribution. Individuals who tend to carry their weight predominantly in their abdomen (central obesity) are at greater risk for developing diabetes, hypertension, cardiovascular disease, and lipid abnormalities, and are referred to as "apples." On the other hand, those whose excess weight is typically distributed in their hips, buttocks, and thighs (peripheral obesity) are described as "pears" (see Figure 3-1). Men more often manifest their obesity as "apples" and thus

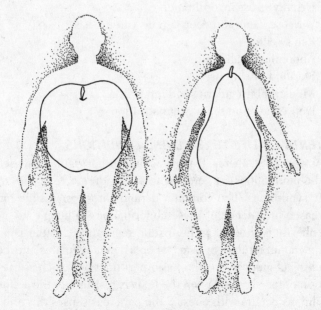

Figure 3-1: "Apples" and "Pears"

have a greater propensity to develop life-threatening complications, whereas women are more frequently "pears."

MEDICAL CONDITIONS ASSOCIATED WITH OBESITY

Potentially Life-Threatening Conditions
Diabetes (type II)
Hypertension
Hyperlipidemia
Cardiovascular disease and stroke
Obstructive sleep apnea—obesity hypoventilation syndrome
Liver disease
Cancer (prostate, colon, breast, uterus)

Lifestyle-Limiting Conditions
Osteoarthritis
Gallstones
Gastroesophageal reflux disease (GERD)
Urinary stress incontinence
Varicose veins and deep venous thrombosis
Leg swelling
Abdominal-wall hernias
Skinfold infections
Menstrual irregularity and infertility
Depression and social stigmatization

POTENTIALLY LIFE-THREATENING CONDITIONS
As a group, diabetes, hypertension, cardiovascular disease, and lipid abnormalities are referred to as "syndrome X" or the "metabolic syndrome." The common denominator responsible for the increased prevalence of these abnormalities in people with central obesity is thought to be insulin resistance. Insulin is a hormone manufactured by the pancreas that regulates the body's handling of glucose. Insulin has other functions, such as the promotion of fat storage. When the body is resistant to the actions of insulin, as occurs with obesity, the pancreas senses this and pro-

duces more insulin in an attempt to overcome the resistance. These high levels of insulin in the blood cause a number of other metabolic abnormalities that result in the components of the syndrome.

Type II Diabetes Mellitus: Diabetes is a disorder of glucose (sugar) metabolism caused by an abnormality in the body's response to insulin, the hormone responsible for the body's handling of glucose. When cells do not respond to insulin properly, the body becomes overloaded with glucose.

Obese people are especially prone to develop type II or adult-onset diabetes. In this type of diabetes, the pancreas makes insulin normally, but the body is resistant to it and does not adequately respond to it. Because people with type II diabetes have enough insulin in their bodies, they only occasionally require synthetic insulin injections. (Type I or juvenile diabetes is usually characterized by a lack of production of insulin by the pancreas. These people have low insulin levels in their blood and almost always require lifelong insulin administration.)

Patients with type II diabetes are at high risk for premature death and disability. Complications of diabetes include cardiovascular disease, hypertension, kidney failure, blindness, and neurological impairment. Approximately 10 million people in the United States suffer from type II diabetes, and over 80 percent of them are obese. Numerous studies have documented that even modest levels of weight loss are associated with significant improvements in glucose control in those with type II diabetes. Several studies by Dr. Walter Pories and his colleagues at East Carolina University have documented rapid and sustained improvement in type II diabetes within days of gastric bypass surgery. The precise mechanism responsible for these changes is unclear; however, it does not appear to be related to weight loss, which is minimal that early post-operatively. These findings challenge traditional views about type II diabetes, and Dr. Pories has even suggested that surgery may become the treatment of choice for patients with type II diabetes and severe obesity.

Hypertension: Hypertension, or high blood pressure, is defined as a blood pressure with either the top (systolic) or the bottom (diastolic) value greater than 140/90 mm Hg. A link between obesity and hypertension exists, with over 30 percent of individuals having a BMI greater than 30 manifesting high blood pressure. Weight loss can usually result in improvement, with people being able to reduce or eliminate their blood-pressure medications.

Hyperlipidemia: Lipids, such as cholesterol and triglycerides, are the various types of fat molecules present in the body. Obese people, especially those with central obesity (the "apples"), are prone to the most dangerous abnormal lipid profile. This pattern, consisting of high LDL-cholesterol ("bad" cholesterol), high triglycerides, and low HDL-cholesterol ("good" cholesterol), is associated with the development of cardiovascular disease. Over 20 percent of individuals with a BMI over 30 have an elevated total serum cholesterol, and over 30 percent have a low HDL-cholesterol level. Significant improvements in these lipid abnormalities can occur with even a modest degree of weight loss.

Cardiovascular Disease: Both coronary artery disease (hardening of the arteries) and stroke are more common in people with obesity. These conditions become more prevalent as BMI increases. Individuals who also have high blood pressure, abnormal lipid profiles, and diabetes are particularly prone to cardiovascular disease and stroke. The prevalence of myocardial infarction (heart attack), stroke, and "sudden-cardiac death" due to a sudden change in the heart's rhythm increase with a higher BMI. Obese patients are at risk for developing cardiomegaly (enlargement of the heart), which increases the chances for congestive heart failure. The benefits of weight loss on reducing cardiovascular risk are less clear-cut because of the contributions of other complicating factors, such as smoking. Presumably, elimination or reduction of these predisposing factors for cardiovascular disease will lower the overall cardiovascular risk, although these measures may be less effective the longer the complications have been present.

Obstructive Sleep Apnea—Obesity Hypoventilation Syndrome (Pickwickian Syndrome): These respiratory problems are among the most dangerous and life-threatening caused by severe obesity. Obstructive sleep apnea is characterized by recurrent periods of apnea (stoppage of breathing) due to obstruction of the upper airway, which results in decreased oxygen levels in the blood and poor sleep patterns. Many affected individuals snore, are drowsy during the day, and develop serious heart problems. The obesity hypoventilation syndrome is a related condition in which the excessive weight of the chest wall and reduced lung size due to compression from the abdomen inhibit effective breathing. This results in decreased oxygen concentration and a buildup of carbon dioxide in the blood, which can cause excessive daytime sleepiness. Obesity hypoventilation syndrome is often accompanied by heart failure. Although each of these problems can occur independently, when they occur together they are referred to as the Pickwickian Syndrome (a term drawn from Charles Dickens' *The Pickwick Papers,* in which his character, a massively obese gentleman, falls asleep during a poker game while holding a winning hand). Both of these conditions can improve dramatically with weight loss.

Liver Disease: Severe obesity is commonly accompanied by increased fat content in the liver, known as nonalcoholic steato-hepatitis (NASH). Previously thought to be innocuous, recent data suggests that a significant number of individuals with NASH may develop permanent changes in liver anatomy, which can, after several years, progress to cirrhosis in some cases. In many cases, weight loss is associated with improvement in NASH.

Cancer: An increased incidence of, and death from, several varieties of cancer has been documented in obese individuals. In men there is a greater risk of developing prostate and colon cancer, and in women, breast, uterine (endometrial), and gallbladder cancer. It is unclear whether this risk decreases with weight loss.

LIFESTYLE-LIMITING CONDITIONS

The obesity-related conditions that limit lifestyle have a greater impact in many instances on the day-to-day lives of the individuals they afflict than do life-threatening illnesses. These maladies can prevent their victims from working, walking, exercising, and can adversely affect their personal relationships and family life.

Osteoarthritis: Joint pain and degenerative arthritis, especially of the lower back, hips, knees, and ankles, are strongly correlated with overweight. These symptoms progress over time and can be completely incapacitating, creating a vicious cycle in which obesity becomes aggravated because of limited ability to engage in physical activity, and limited activity causes more weight gain. Although symptoms of pain and inflammation can improve with weight loss, the physical changes in the joints produced over time are often irreversible, leading to permanent disability. This engenders an enormous cost to society in terms of days lost from work, medications (analgesics and anti-inflammatory drugs), and surgery.

Gallstones: The gallbladder is located in the right upper portion of the abdomen, beneath the liver. Its function is to store bile, which is made in the liver and released into the intestine to assist with digestion. Gallstones result from a chemical imbalance in the bile in which bile-salt crystals coalesce to form stones. These stones can become lodged in the "neck" (narrow portion) of the gallbladder, causing pain (especially after eating greasy food), inflammation, and infection. The only reliable treatment for gallstones is removal of the gallbladder (a procedure called cholecystectomy). The risk of developing gallstones increases with weight, rising to approximately 25 percent in women and 10 percent in men with a BMI above 40. In addition, rapid weight loss is also associated with a greater tendency to develop symptomatic gallstones. Since treatment of symptomatic gallstones requires surgery, the cost in terms of money and time lost from work is considerable.

Gastroesophageal Reflux Disease (GERD): A certain degree of reflux (backflow of acid stomach contents into the esophagus, or food pipe) is normal; however, excessive reflux is typically due to an abnormally loose muscle at the junction of the esophagus and stomach. Reflux is usually manifested by heartburn, which is aggravated by lying down or bending over. Acid reflux can also lead to choking on stomach acid that is aspirated into the lungs, pneumonia, and cancer of the esophagus. The increase in pressure within the abdomen due to obesity is partly responsible for the higher incidence of reflux. The cost of drugs frequently prescribed for treatment (similar to those used for stomach ulcers), diagnostic studies (upper-GI series and endoscopy), and occasionally surgery is high. Symptoms typically improve with weight loss.

Urinary Stress Incontinence: Although most common in women after childbirth, obesity increases the propensity for developing urinary stress incontinence by increasing the pressure on the bladder from within the abdomen. These embarrassing symptoms can be mild, with minimal leakage of urine when laughing, sneezing, or coughing, or more disabling, preventing people from going out in public. In the absence of significant sustained weight loss, surgery is often required to control the problem, but the failure rate is high.

Venous Disease and Leg Swelling: Chronic venous disease refers to the formation of blood clots (deep venous thrombosis) and subsequent damage to the valves in the leg veins, which prevents the backflow of blood. Obesity predisposes people to venous disease because of the decreased mobility and greater resistance to blood return from the legs to the heart; their increased body weight leads to stagnation of blood and clotting. The most serious problem associated with deep venous thrombosis is pulmonary embolism, which occurs when a portion of the clot breaks off and lodges in the lungs and can be fatal. Once clots have formed, damage to the veins often results, producing chronic leg ulcers and changes in skin color and vein thickness. People with severe ulcers cannot participate in normal recreational or work activities. Although weight loss can lead to improvement in symptoms, once changes in the veins or skin occur, they are permanent. Leg swelling (edema) often happens as the result of an accumulation of excess fluid in the legs, which are the most dependent parts of the body. The swelling is aggravated by the excess weight in the abdomen, which increases the pressure on the veins of the legs and impairs the return of blood and fluid from the legs to the heart.

Abdominal-wall Hernias: Obesity is associated with an elevation in abdominal pressure (the pressure within the belly). This increase is often exerted directly on the abdominal wall. If a weakness in the wall is present, the chronic increase in pressure can create a "hole" in the abdominal wall (hernia), through which fat or intestine can protrude. Most hernias only enlarge with time and need to be repaired surgically.

Skinfold Infections: Occasionally, the skin of the lower abdominal wall droops down to the groin. This hanging portion (pannus) is difficult to clean and perspires easily, often becoming chafed and infected with fungus or bacteria, causing cellulitis.

Menstrual Irregularity and Infertility: A normal menstrual cycle requires an intact hormonal system, with well-regulated proportions of estrogen, progesterone, and testosterone. In obese women, the excess fat can bind these hormones, leading to amenorrhea (absence of a period) or menstrual irregularity and infertility. These problems often resolve with weight loss.

Depression and Social Stigmatization: Obese individuals face discrimination in several areas, including school, work, and the social arena. Obese students receive lower grades and have lower acceptance rates to colleges. Workers who are obese have greater difficulty finding jobs and higher rates of unemployment. Obese people are also considered undesirable socially and romantically in our society. They're made the butt of jokes and are ridiculed in public. Because they interact less with others socially and because there is so much prejudice directed at them, they have fewer marriage opportunities. Discriminatory attitudes toward the obese among health-care providers have also been documented. Although studies have failed to substantiate that any psychological problems are unique to obese patients, societal prejudices contribute to feelings of low self-esteem and depression. Not surprisingly, psychological issues often improve with weight loss.

Most patients perceive obesity as a huge liability. One study revealed that individuals who successfully lost weight and kept it off would rather suffer from a disability, such as diabetes, dyslexia, blindness, or an amputation, than return to being morbidly obese. Given the hypothetical choice, all said they preferred to be normal weight rather than a morbidly obese multimillionaire.

The risks of representative co-morbid conditions in relation to BMI for men and women are shown in Table 3-2. Table 3-3 shows the actual prevalence of obesity-related co-morbid medical conditions in my own practice.

Table 3-2: Health Risk and BMI
(from World Health Organization)

Men

Condition	Prevalence—Percent			
	Normal	Obese	Severely Obese	Morbidly Obese
Type II diabetes mellitus	2.0	4.9	10.1	10.7
Coronary heart disease	8.8	9.6	14.0	16.0
Hypertension	23.5	34.2	49.0	64.5
Osteoarthritis	2.6	4.6	4.7	10.0

Women

Condition	Prevalence—Percent			
	Normal	Obese	Severely Obese	Morbidly Obese
Type II diabetes mellitus	2.4	7.1	7.2	19.9
Coronary heart disease	6.9	11.1	12.6	19.2
Hypertension	23.3	38.8	48.0	63.1
Osteoarthritis	5.2	8.5	9.9	17.2

Table 3-3: Frequency of Obesity-Related Medical Conditions in Patients Treated Surgically

Condition	Frequency (percent)
Potentially Life-Threatening Conditions	
Diabetes (type II)	18
Hypertension	47
Hyperlipidemia	36
Cardiovascular disease	19
Obstructive sleep apnea—obesity hypoventilation syndrome	17
Liver disease	90
Lifestyle-Limiting Conditions	
Osteoarthritis or joint pain	81
Gallstones	32
Gastroesophageal reflux	21
Urinary stress incontinence	45
Varicose veins and deep venous thrombosis	23
Leg swelling	44
Abdominal-wall hernias and skinfold infections	21
Secondary amenorrhea	17
Depression (treated)	23

4

WHY CONSIDER WEIGHT LOSS SURGERY?

My family thought that the idea of surgery to correct obesity was nuts—but I did my research and I knew it was my last hope.

Leora M., 37, 347 lbs. pre-op; 212 lbs. 20 months post-op

I watched my best friend go through WLS and I saw how it changed her life. Once she was brave enough, I followed her lead.

Natalie G., 41, 294 lbs. pre-op; 168 lbs. 4 years post-op

The field of weight loss surgery, also known as bariatric surgery (from the Greek *baros*—weight—and *iatrike*—treatment), has existed for almost forty years. Operations that induce weight loss involve making modifications to the stomach, intestines, or both, altering the amount of food consumed and the number of calories that can be absorbed. These anatomic and metabolic changes result in substantial weight loss, which can be maintained over many years.

Bariatric surgical procedures differ from liposuction and other cosmetic procedures because they do not involve the removal of fat deposits and are not primarily designed to improve body contour and appearance. Liposuction and cosmetic-surgery procedures improve physical appearance by removing localized areas of excessive fat tissue and reshaping the body contour. Liposuction does not produce any significant amount of weight loss or alter eating, absorption, or the body's metabolism in any way.

Why consider weight loss surgery? Because it works! Surgical treatment of clinically severe obesity is the ONLY treatment that predictably and reliably produces significant and sustained weight loss.

NONSURGICAL TREATMENTS FOR OBESITY

Treatment of obesity is generally divided into medical and surgical remedies. Medical approaches usually consist of dietary and/or drug therapy in combination with behavior modification and exercise. Surgery is reserved for patients with clinically severe or morbid obesity.

Most Common Weight Loss Approaches

Diets: The most popular type of diet is the balanced-deficit diet. These diets call for a reasonable reduction in calorie intake (between 1,200 and 1,800 calories per day) while maintaining a normal distribution of calories from protein, carbohydrate, and fat. Low-calorie diets (800 to 1,200 calories per day) are used in moderately overweight persons (BMI between 27 and 30), with very low-calorie (below 800 calories per day) diets reserved for individuals with a BMI above 30. Both low- and very low-calorie diets consist of an active weight loss period of three to four months, followed by a prolonged maintenance phase. During the active phase, patients on low-calorie diets typically lose 20 to 40 pounds (10 to 15 percent of body weight) and those on very low-calorie diets lose 30 to 60 pounds (15 to 20 percent of body weight). The weight loss tends to be rapid at first but then tapers off over time, eventually reaching a plateau.

During this energy-deficient period, the body is in a state of semi-starvation. It adapts by decreasing its energy consumption as much as 30 percent and utilizing stored internal energy—carbohydrate initially, then protein, and ultimately fat. This use of energy is analogous to the way a family might conserve money by using all of the food in the pantry before buying more food. These changes in the body's ability to use stored energy compensate for the decrease in food intake and prevent weight loss.

These compensatory mechanisms make losing weight by dieting difficult.

Exercise: In an effort to overcome the compensatory changes designed to prevent weight loss, exercise is commonly promoted as a necessary component of any weight loss regimen. Moderate exercise, per se, is ineffective as a means of achieving weight loss. Numerous studies evaluating exercise alone, in the absence of dietary restriction, show that it produces little if any weight loss. It does appear, however, that exercise is an excellent way to promote preservation of muscle mass during dieting. Thus, exercise is more important in maintaining weight loss than in achieving it. When exercise is combined with dieting, it is probably better that it be done early in the morning so that any increase in metabolic rate that does occur can be sustained throughout the day.

Behavior Modification: Behavior modification involves making permanent lifestyle changes that promote healthier eating habits. It contributes to improved weight loss and maintenance when compared to diets alone. However, it is often difficult to get patients to continue returning to the dietitian or therapist in order to obtain the necessary counseling and reinforcement to sustain these changes. People find it hard to make a lifetime commitment and tend to revert to their old eating habits.

Drug Treatment: Drug treatment has also produced limited success but has been subjected to intense scrutiny because of public and regulatory concerns over the safety of long-term treatment. This is particularly problematic because obesity is a chronic disorder. So in order to be effective in patients who are severely overweight, drugs must be given continuously, as in the treatment of other chronic diseases such as high blood pressure or diabetes. In the past, these amphetamine-like drugs were addictive and illegal. Newer, nonaddictive drugs are now available. However, serious concerns about their safety have been raised when they were used for even moderate lengths of time, let alone for long-term treatment. Most studies have shown that weight loss with drugs usually peaks at about 45 pounds after treatment for three to six months, with most patients regaining their weight when treatment is halted.

THE PROBLEM WITH NONSURGICAL TREATMENTS

The difficulty associated with obesity treatment is clearly reflected by its high rates of failure and weight regain. The best data available on the effectiveness of diets, behavior modification, and exercise still demonstrate that over 90 percent of patients will regain over 90 percent of their lost weight within three years. Little scientific data is available documenting the effectiveness and safety of most commercial weight loss regimens. Medically supervised weight loss programs, usually consisting of very low-calorie diets in combination with behavior modification and exercise, have met with modest success but still suffer from a high degree of weight regain. In the morbidly obese, the effectiveness of these modes of treatment is even less. Regarding the value of nonsurgical approaches to weight loss in severely overweight individuals, the National Institutes of Health's *Technology Assessment of Methods of Voluntary Weight Loss* (1992) stated: *Although acceptable weight reduction may be achieved, a major drawback to the nonsurgical approach is failure to maintain reduced body weight in the vast majority of patients.*

MY LIFE ON DIETS

Erica Manfred, 57, 255 lbs. pre-op; 180 lbs. 2 years post-op

As a lifelong dieter, I can attest to the failure of one diet after another. As a teenager, I was put on a diet by a doctor who gave me amphetamines. I lost 30 pounds, but I was so edgy I couldn't sleep. When I stopped taking the pills, I gained all the weight back. A lifetime of dieting followed. I tried the Atkins Diet, Weight Watchers, the Scarsdale Diet, the banana and grapefruit diet, Jenny Craig, liquid diets, and others I can't even remember. Always losing initially and then regaining what I'd lost plus a few extra pounds. Finally I gave up, deciding that I would stay fat and accept myself.

While attending compulsive-eating groups led by various therapists, I found out why diets didn't work for me. In addition to slowing the metabolism, which makes it more difficult to lose weight, every diet led me to manifest an equal and opposite reaction—a binge. As soon as I was restricted and denied certain foods, they became the most desirable. I found myself in front of the refrigerator at midnight, gorging on forbidden goodies.

Over the years I spent in these groups, I saw many smaller women successfully deal with their compulsive eating, while I failed. I could not quell my compulsive eating without extra help. Finally, I developed diabetes when I was 40. The prospect of a shortened life span with horrible complications caused by this disease eventually led me to WLS.

WHO SAYS SURGERY WORKS?

My husband and I both had WLS, and believe me, it works. We are now able to take walks together, sit comfortably in movie seats, and travel without making all sorts of complicated arrangements.

Doreen, 43, 334 lbs. pre-op; 198 lbs. 4 years post-op
Robbie B., 46, 422 lbs. pre-op; 287 lbs. 4 years post-op

I used to weigh 300 pounds and now I weigh 200. It makes a difference. I can wear fashionable clothing and I feel great. I don't quite understand why, but gastric bypass really worked when everything else failed.

Georgann D., 34, 302 lbs. pre-op; 201 lbs. 18 months post-op

In 1991, the National Institutes of Health (NIH) convened a Consensus Development Conference to evaluate gastrointestinal surgery for severe obesity. For two days, experts from around the world discussed various aspects of clinically severe obesity and its surgical treatment and presented the results of their research and personal experiences to an impartial panel. The panel then analyzed the material and issued its report, concluding that:

> *the surgical procedures currently in use are capable of inducing significant weight loss in severely obese patients, which in turn has been associated with amelioration of most of the co-morbid conditions that have been studied.*

Since the NIH Consensus Development Conference, several other health organizations have also addressed the surgical treatment of severe obesity while developing their own guidelines for the treatment of this disease. In 1996, Shape Up America! and the American Obesity Association formulated a joint set of *Guidances for the Treatment of Adult Obesity*. In 1997, both the American Heart Association and the American Dietetic Association published position papers addressing the surgical treatment of severe obesity. Subsequently, in 1998, the World Health Organization published a report entitled *Obesity: Preventing and Managing the Global Epidemic*. In late 1998, the National Institutes of Health performed a thorough analysis of the published literature on the treatment of obesity and categorized the results based on the quality of the research. The NIH then issued a set of comprehensive *Clinical Guidelines on the Identification, Evaluation and Treatment of Overweight and Obesity in Adults*. In 2000, these guidelines were updated in *The Practical Guide: Identification, Evaluation and Treatment of Overweight and Obesity*. In each of these analyses, surgical treatment of clinically severe obesity was assessed and subsequently endorsed. A summary of statements from these organizations endorsing the surgical treatment of clinically severe obesity is presented in Table 4-1. The general guidelines currently in use in clinical practice are summarized in Table 4-2.

Table 4-1: Summary of Statements Endorsing Surgical Treatment of Clinically Severe Obesity

National Institutes of Health Consensus Development Conference (1991)

> . . . *the surgical procedures currently in use [such as Roux-en-Y gastric bypass and vertical banded gastroplasty] are capable of inducing significant weight loss in severely obese patients, which in turn has been associated with amelioration of most of the co-morbid conditions that have been studied . . . while limited success has been achieved by a variety of techniques that include medically supervised weight loss and intensive behavior modification . . . a major drawback of the non-surgical ap-*

proach is failure to maintain reduced body weight in the vast majority of patients.

Shape Up America!/American Obesity Association: *Guidances for the Treatment of Adult Obesity (1996)*

Surgical treatment for obesity should be considered for patients with a BMI above 40 or a BMI above 35 with co-morbidities or other risk factors.

American Heart Association Science Advisory and Coordinating Committee: *Obesity and Heart Disease (1997)*

When the BMI is above 35 and co-morbidities exist, gastrointestinal surgery becomes a consideration. When the BMI is >40, surgery is the treatment of choice. The experience of the surgeon and type of operation chosen predict outcome. In general, a Roux-en-Y gastric bypass is superior to gastric plication [stomach stapling].

American Dietetic Association: Position Paper on Weight Management (1997)

Surgical treatment of obesity should be limited to patients with a BMI over 40 or BMI over 35 and severe co-morbid conditions related to the obesity. Roux-en-Y gastric bypass and vertical banded gastroplasty are the most commonly performed and widely accepted procedures currently in use.

Seventy percent of patients maintain a loss of 50 percent of their initial excess weight for five years. Improvements in cardiovascular functioning, lipid profile, sleep apnea, physical activity, and work abilities have been reported.

World Health Organization: *Obesity: Preventing and Managing the Global Epidemic (1998)*

Surgery is now considered to be the most effective way of reducing weight, and maintaining weight loss, in severely (BMI above 35) and very severely obese (BMI above 40) subjects. On a kg/weight loss basis, surgical treatment has been estimated after four years to be less expensive than any other treatment.

NIH, National Heart Lung and Blood Institute: *Clinical Guidelines on the Identification, Evaluation and Treatment of Overweight and Obesity in Adults—The Evidence Report (1998)*

Gastrointestinal surgery can result in substantial weight loss, and therefore is an available weight loss option for well-informed and motivated patients with BMI above 40 or BMI above 35, who have co-morbid conditions and acceptable operative risks.

NIH, National Heart Lung and Blood Institute, North American Association for the Study of Obesity: *The Practical Guide— Identification, Evaluation, and Treatment of Overweight and Obesity in Adults (2000)*

Weight loss surgery provides medically significant sustained weight loss for more than five years in most patients. Surgery is an option for well-informed and motivated patients who have clinically severe obesity (BMI >40) or a BMI >35 and serious co-morbid conditions.

Table 4-2: Guidelines for the Surgical Treatment of Clinically Severe Obesity

Patients must have a BMI over 40 or a BMI over 35 with severe associated medical problems;

Patients should have failed or be likely to fail at dietary and/or drug treatment;

Patients must have no contraindications to surgery, such as uncontrolled binge-eating disorder, anorexia/bulimia, terminal malignancy, etc.;

Patients must be able to comprehend the nature of the procedure and provide voluntary informed consent; and

Patients must be willing to commit to long-term follow-up.

5

A TOUGH DECISION TO MAKE

Here is why one man finally turned to WLS:

William J., 55, 377 lbs. pre-op; 300 lbs. 6 months post-op

For most of my life, I lived in Nashville, Tennessee. My mother was a traditional southern cook who raised me on fried catfish and chicken, biscuits dripping with butter, and mashed potatoes smothered in gravy. Peggy and I married young, and she took over where my mother left off, plying me with down-home cooking. The funny thing is that Peggy never really ate what she cooked. She picked at the food on her plate, and I scarfed down her leftovers. My dear wife stayed thin and I got bigger and bigger—sort of like Jack Sprat and his wife. As a result of the efforts of the women in my life, some bad genes, and a lack of self-control, I was fat—250 pounds or so.

Then my company transferred me to New York City. Peggy and I bought a small co-op on the Upper West Side of Manhattan, and it was there I really started to eat. Right in my own backyard there was Thai, Japanese, Cuban, Ethiopian, Italian, Mexican, and Jewish food. I was thrilled to experience the cuisines of the world without even walking more than a few blocks from home. I fell in love with hot-pastrami sandwiches, rice and beans, knishes and tempura.

Each morning I avoided looking at the scale, until one day I shored up my courage and found that it tipped at over 300 pounds. I knew that I was killing myself by eating. Over the past several years,

I had developed diabetes, high blood pressure, and high cholesterol. My legs swelled after walking short distances, I suffered from chronic heartburn, and I had arthritis in my joints. One night I had an angina attack and Peggy had to rush me to the hospital. Needless to say, we were both terrified. Although it wasn't a heart attack, my doctor saw the beginnings of coronary artery disease. All the grease-laden food was settling in my arteries. I knew that my health was declining and I was determined to do something about it.

For several months I was a regular at Weight Watchers meetings. I measured and weighed everything that went into my mouth. I began to lose small amounts of weight. Then Peggy and I took a European vacation, and I ate my way through Paris, Rome, and London. It took no more than a week for me to gain back every ounce I had worked so hard to shed. I came back from our trip angry with myself and more discouraged than ever.

Unpacking my suitcase, I realized that I needed to take more pills than the average 55-year-old man. In fact, I was taking more drugs than my 85-year-old father. I had one medication for my blood pressure, two others for diabetes, and on and on. I didn't like to admit it, but all these pills were having adverse effects on me. My hair was thinning from one of them, my libido was waning from another, and my energy level was declining from yet another. I knew I couldn't keep going on the way I was.

A friend of mine from work was trying Optifast and having good results. I decided to jump on that bandwagon. I stayed on that diet for a few months and lost quite a bit of weight, but I felt miserable. Food was one of my greatest pleasures, and I wanted to taste something, I wanted something to chew. I knew that I couldn't stay on this program forever, it just wasn't normal. I stuck it out for a while, but as soon as I went back to real food, I gained all of the weight back and then some. It's humiliating to confess this, but I was 377 pounds.

Peggy made me an appointment with a registered dietitian named Kathy at a hospital known for the treatment of obesity. Kathy took one look at me and my medical records and said, "We need to talk seriously about your health." Then she told me about WLS. Naturally, I had heard of it before, but I always thought it was something kind of on the fringe of traditional medicine. She said that it is the only proven effective and safe method of achieving and sustaining weight loss in the morbidly obese and that it was the only way of improving some of my medical problems. Before I had a chance to think about what she had told me, she was scheduling me for an appointment with the surgeon associated with their program. Clearly, she felt strongly about what I should do.

I went home, talked the situation over with Peggy, and did a little of my own research on the Internet. Although Kathy was sure about what course I should take, this was not an easy decision for me. I discovered that what Kathy told me was true—surgery was my last best hope of regaining my health. Peggy arranged to take the day off from work and she accompanied me for my surgical consultation. I hit it off with my surgeon right from the start, because he willingly answered all of my questions without pulling any punches. He told me about all of the risks involved in having the operation and all the risks involved in not having it. I wanted my life back. Peggy and I were at the point where our kids were finally independent and we were living in the most exciting city in the world. I just wanted to enjoy our precious time together.

Actually making the appointment for the operation was a little frightening. Rearranging meetings at the office and canceling appointments forced me to realize that this process was going to change my life. The first thing I needed to do was to make the commitment to put my life on hold for a while. Again, I questioned if I was doing the right thing, but ultimately I figured it was a small price to pay in order to buy me a few extra years on this earth.

The night before my surgery, my grown son and two daughters surprised me by flying in from Nashville. Seeing them bolstered my confidence that this was the right choice and distracted me from my fears. I was so happy that they would be able to sit with Peggy in the surgical waiting room during the operation and sleep in the apartment with her while I was in the hospital. The time between checking in and actually being brought into the operating room seemed short, because my younger daughter entertained us with a bunch of jokes she had gotten on her e-mail.

It took only an hour from start to finish for the operation that changed my life forever. I had some pain that first night. Luckily, the pain was not as bad as I had feared, since the morphine didn't agree with me and I vomited several times and just felt horrible. They gave me medication for the nausea and the next day I was able to get some rest. I was actually ready to go home on the second day after surgery, but they kept me an extra day to rearrange my diabetes medications. By the time I went home, I was eating pureed foods and taking only small amounts of oral pain medication.

It's been only six months since my surgery, and the results are amazing. I hate to sound melodramatic, but this operation is really a miracle. I'm not thin, but I have lost 75 pounds. More importantly, my diabetes, high blood pressure, and leg swelling are cured. There is improvement in my coronary artery disease, my arthritis, and my heartburn. I never thought it would be possible, but now I take fewer pills than Dad. The side effects I had from my pills are starting to dissipate. Peggy and I still eat out often, but instead of eating an entire pastrami on rye, I eat a quarter of a sandwich. I don't indulge in fried catfish when we go back down south, because it no longer agrees with me. I've lost my taste for sweets, a frequent side effect of gastric bypass, which makes passing up the dessert cart much easier. If I overeat, I don't feel well, and that also helps keep me on the straight and narrow path. The most dramatic change in my relationship with my wife has occurred as a result of this operation. Now Peggy sometimes steals leftover food from my plate instead of the other way around—simply amazing!

No one turns to WLS as an initial solution to weight loss. Usually, it is the last resort after numerous other options have been explored, attempted, and then failed. Typically, patients have tried a variety of diets, including commercial programs (Weight Watchers, Jenny Craig, Richard Simmons), self-administered programs (Slim-Fast, Overeaters Anonymous), medically supervised programs (Optifast, Nutrisystems), fad diets (Atkins Diet, cabbage diet, grapefruit diet), over-the-counter drugs (Dexatrim, Fat Burners), prescription drugs (fen-phen, Redux, Meridia, Xenical), and exercise and behavior modification, all with varying degrees of success. Many patients have spent thousands of dollars to lose hundreds of pounds, only to regain them, and more.

The majority of individuals seeking surgical relief have suffered from obesity for most of their lives. A minority became obese as adults, after childbirth, as a result of an injury that severely limited their physical ability, or in conjunction with an emotionally traumatic event. Virtually all candidates for surgery believe that they have exhausted all available resources before considering surgery.

By the time obese individuals decide upon surgical treatment, they have thought long and hard about the effects of severe obesity on their lives. They have considered their options, agonized over the decision, and often endured many negative comments from uninformed and skeptical family members and friends. Nevertheless, these patients have concluded that surgery is the appropriate option for them. It is anything but taking the easy way out.

The toll morbid obesity takes on its sufferers is incalculable. In addition to the inevitable health problems that come with severe obesity, those who finally turn to surgery often have heartrending stories of rejection, humiliation, and misery. It is a testament to the human spirit that they chose to survive and eventually to thrive after WLS. Unfortunately, obese people are subjected to a unique form of prejudice because our society assumes that we could lose weight if only we tried hard enough.

6

GETTING STARTED: SELECTING A SURGEON

There is a saying that when purchasing real estate, the three most important factors to consider are: 1) location, 2) location, and 3) location. In the same way, the three most important factors to consider in selecting a surgeon for bariatric surgery are: 1) commitment, 2) commitment, and 3) commitment.

Obesity is a chronic disease, and individuals who suffer from clinically severe obesity will continue to do so, even after successful WLS. None of the operations currently in use return patients to their ideal body weight. Rather, after successful WLS, most people go from being a lot overweight to being a lot less overweight, but the vast majority will still be overweight. For this reason, patients suffering from severe obesity need long-term follow-up from their surgeon and other health-care providers.

WLS has become a highly specialized area, with only a small group of surgeons nationwide committed to it. In their hands, WLS can be done safely and successfully. However, most surgeons are not interested in caring for severely overweight patients. They fear that the surgery is technically difficult, fraught with complications, and many do not want to make the commitment to follow the patients long-term. In addition, most successful surgical weight loss programs provide nutritional counseling at post-operative visits, and many sponsor patient support groups after surgery. These services are time-consuming and expensive, and many surgeons do not have the resources to provide them.

Because most physicians, especially family practitioners and internists, are unfamiliar with WLS, it is critical for the surgeons involved to be dedicated to providing long-term care, since many problems that may arise, like iron or vitamin deficiency, will not be identified otherwise. Many general surgeons are unfamiliar with the technical details and post-operative complications that can arise after WLS. Therefore, they are often reluctant to treat even routine general surgical problems in patients who have had WLS.

Most well-trained, board-certified general surgeons are competent to perform WLS. If they brushed up on the most current techniques or spent some time training with an experienced bariatric surgeon, they could master the technical aspects within a reasonable amount of time. However, it is the surgeon's commitment to treating obesity that ultimately determines the success of his or her patients.

The explosion of laparoscopic surgery has brought up concerns, because it has been applied to bariatric surgical procedures. Latham Flanagan, M.D., president of the American Society for Bariatric Surgery (ASBS) from 1999 to 2000, addressed this issue in his August 1999 Letter from the President to the ASBS membership.

> *The core issue . . . is that surgeons who are not aware of the principles of bariatric surgery are taking up this operation. The temptation is particularly strong in laparoscopic surgery where the race for reputation has carried surgeons to explore the limits of what can be done through a laparoscope. . . . The problem we face is that there are some individuals who are enamored with the technology of performing bariatric surgery through the laparoscope, but are not particularly interested in the complex and long-term relationship to the bariatric surgical patient that is so necessary for success in achieving profound and lasting weight loss. . . .*

I fear that, over time, patients will be lost to follow-up, and should they develop complications, the requisite expertise needed to properly care for them will not be readily available. Thus, it is this commitment to becoming knowledgeable in all aspects of WLS, both before and after surgery, that is the most critical criterion for selecting a surgeon and a WLS program.

GUIDELINES FOR SELECTING A SURGEON

Many factors enter into the decision. For some, the choice will be based upon medical-school degrees, residency training, and number of operations performed, while for others it will be based upon the rapport they establish with the surgeon. There is no foolproof method. Some of the items that can affect the decision are listed below:

Professional Qualifications

Where he or she attended college and medical school will offer little information concerning competence as a surgeon. Where they received their surgical training (residency and/or fellowship) could be useful to someone knowledgeable in the field but will not be helpful to most laypeople. Therefore, the most useful information will be whether the surgeon is board-certified in general surgery. Board certification indicates that the surgeon has successfully completed an accredited residency training program in surgery (usually at least five years) and passed an examination administered by the American Board of Surgery. This is the highest standard currently available.

Beyond board certification, many surgeons belong to various professional societies. One of the most prestigious is membership in the Fellowship of the American College of Surgeons, denoted by the initials FACS. In addition, there are a number of professional societies devoted to specific areas of interest. The ASBS and the International Federation for the Surgery of Obesity are solely devoted to WLS. Other professional societies with related interests include the Society for Surgery of the Alimentary Tract, the North American Association for the Study of Obesity, the American Society for Clinical Nutrition, and the American Obesity Association. Membership in one or more of these societies is an indication of the person's interest and commitment to the field of obesity and its treatment.

Experience

Many studies have documented lower complication rates among surgeons who perform a particular procedure more frequently. How many procedures it takes to become proficient in bariatric surgery is difficult to know. The frequency with which one performs weight loss procedures is more significant than the absolute number done. A surgeon performing about fifty or more per year should have the requisite technical skills and experience.

For surgeons performing laparoscopic bariatric surgery, it is necessary that they have experience with advanced laparoscopic techniques as well as with open bariatric surgery. There are occasions when it is necessary to convert a laparoscopic procedure into an open procedure.

Personality and Bedside Manner

These areas are variable and difficult to judge objectively. Their significance varies greatly among patients—some want the "most qualified and expert," while others prefer someone who is "warm and easy to talk to."

The surgeon should be available and should be willing and able to discuss the recommended procedure with you. He or she should be able to describe the procedure, the anticipated hospital course, risks and potential complications, and long-term results. Unwillingness to do so or to answer other questions should raise a concern.

LOCATING A BARIATRIC SURGEON

Most bariatric-surgery practices in the United States grow primarily via patient-to-patient referrals. This differs from other types of medical and surgical practices in which the practitioners also obtain large numbers of patients through physician referrals. Due to the lack of knowledge about—and prejudice against—severe obesity and its surgical treatment in the medical community, patients cannot rely on referrals from their family doctor or other physicians. Therefore, many patients will identify a surgeon based on the advice of an acquaintance who already had WLS. Others may ask their personal physicians about potential surgeons, but their physicians may not know whether these surgeons have any interest or expertise in bariatric surgery. Another useful source of information is the American Society for Bariatric Surgery (www.asbs.org), which maintains an active geographic directory.

Finding a surgeon close to you will make follow-up care easier. There is really no substitute for, or parallel in medicine to, the relationship between a surgeon and a patient on whom he or she has operated. Many surgeons tend to become possessive of their patients because of the unique nature of the surgeon–patient connection and the personal responsibility they bear for their patients' outcomes. Similarly, surgeons may be reluctant to assume the care of patients operated on elsewhere by others because they lack the intimate, firsthand knowledge about the actual procedure performed. This is especially true if complications of the original procedure arise, when the details of the procedure can be critical to correctly deciphering the problem.

Unfortunately, because there are a limited number of surgeons performing bariatric surgery (the current membership of the ASBS is about 750), the nearest qualified surgeon may be several hours away. Since follow-up with the surgeon is necessary, each candidate should be prepared to make the commitment to return for follow-up at regular intervals. In these situations, arrangements can be made to have some of the follow-up visits provided by local practitioners who can work closely with your surgeon. However, it is advisable to maintain contact with your surgeon and keep him or her informed of your progress.

Commercial WLS treatment facilities typically advertise in the press and media and accept patients for treatment from far away. In these situations, patients often assume that they can get effective follow-up care from a local family physician or internist and that surgical complications will not arise. However, this is not always the case. Should complications arise, it may be impossible to fly back to the surgeon in a timely manner, leaving the care to unknowledgeable individuals. It may also be difficult to enlist the help of a local surgeon with expertise in bariatric surgery if he or she is aware that you chose to go out of town for your primary operation.

Research and select your surgeon carefully, based upon what

best fits your needs. If you do have to travel any significant distance, set up a relationship beforehand with a local physician who is willing to communicate with your surgeon about any complications that might arise.

THE TEAM AND THE HOSPITAL

No (wo)man is an island. This adage is very applicable to WLS. Although selection of the surgeon is important, it really takes an entire team to effectively care for patients having WLS, before, during, and after the actual operation. For instance, even with a highly qualified registered dietitian to counsel patients post-operatively, there is information and expertise that a surgeon possesses that will never be known by a dietitian, just as there is knowledge about nutrition and feeding that will never be known by a surgeon. These two roles are complementary; one cannot serve as a substitute for the other.

Ideally, a team of health-care professionals—including physicians, registered dietitians, mental-health professionals, nurses, and operating-room staff—is involved in patient care. Although not every member of the team needs to be involved in every case, it is important that there is a group of people with the necessary skills and expertise to work together to assist in the care of patients as needed.

Although most physicians—especially those who serve as consultants, such as endocrinologists, pulmonologists, or cardiologists—do not limit their practices to the treatment of obesity, additional expertise is acquired by caring for a large number of obese patients. In the case of the anesthesiologist, a critical member of the operating team, the level of skill required to successfully intubate (place the breathing tube in the windpipe) and manage severely obese patients in the operating room improves with experience.

Many of these team members will be totally dedicated to the care of WLS patients. For example, many programs have full-time dietitians devoted to the care of weight loss patients. These dietitians may be involved in pre-operative evaluation and counseling, teaching in the hospital before discharge, and post-operative evaluation and counseling. Many programs also offer support groups after surgery, and the dietitian may play a role as a facilitator or educator.

The hospital may also demonstrate its commitment to the care of WLS patients in a number of ways. Patients may be housed on a particular unit before and after surgery and be cared for by specially trained nurses who are knowledgeable of and sensitive to the unique needs of severely overweight individuals. The patient-care unit may be specifically reengineered to better accommodate large patients, with customized furniture, enlarged toilets and shower facilities, and gowns that maintain dignity and modesty. There may be a designated operating room and staff assigned to these cases, so that skilled personnel and the appropriate equipment are always available.

Each of these examples demonstrates a certain level of commitment to the care of severely obese patients. While none of them is critical to the successful performance of WLS, each contributes to making an otherwise unpleasant and frightening experience somewhat more tolerable.

7

THE OPERATIONS

I had a gastric bypass because, after talking it over with my surgeon, it seemed as if that was the safest, most effective way to go for me.

Ted J., 51, 292 lbs. pre-op; 172 lbs. 6 years post-op

The field of bariatric surgery has been evolving for several decades. The concept of using gastrointestinal surgery to control obesity grew out of results of operations for cancer or peptic-ulcer disease in which large portions of the stomach or small intestine were removed. Because patients undergoing these procedures tended to lose a great deal of weight after surgery, some surgeons adapted these operations to treat severe obesity.

Operative procedures have been refined as knowledge about obesity, nutrition, and the consequences of different surgical techniques has increased. Each technique entails risks and benefits. The risks are the complications that result from the procedure, while the benefits relate to the amount of weight lost, reduction of co-morbid conditions, and improvements in lifestyle. Usually, the procedures that produce the greatest weight loss are associated with higher operative risk and more complications. The best operation for any individual involves a careful analysis balancing all of the risks and benefits.

STRUCTURE AND FUNCTION OF THE GASTROINTESTINAL TRACT

In order to understand the different operations that are performed for the treatment of obesity, it is necessary to be familiar with the anatomy and function of the gastrointestinal (GI) tract.

The GI tract, shown schematically in Figure 7-1, is essentially a tube measuring about thirty feet, extending from the mouth to the anus. Along its path, it is divided into specialized portions, known as the esophagus, stomach, small intestine, and large intestine (or colon). Each of these sections has a unique structure and function involved in the transportation, absorption, and digestion of nutrients.

The *esophagus* is a narrow, straight tube connecting the throat to the stomach, whose primary function is to serve as a passageway for food. No digestion or absorption occurs there. The esophagus is separated from the stomach by a muscle, the lower esophageal sphincter, which allows food to enter and, when functioning normally, prevents stomach contents from flowing back upward and causing "acid reflux" and heartburn.

The *stomach* is the site of the initial breakdown of food. As food enters the stomach, it comes into contact with acid and digestive enzymes (proteins that facilitate digestion) that are secreted by the stomach. The presence of food in the stomach stimulates other parts of the GI tract to release hormones to assist in other aspects of digestion. The stomach wall is muscular and churns the food until it is transformed into a thick "mush" (chyme) that can be transported into the small intestine. Additionally, the stomach secretes a chemical (intrinsic factor) that assists in the absorption of vitamin B_{12}.

The partially digested food is squeezed out of the stomach through an opening known as the pylorus into the *duodenum,* which is the first part of the small intestine. The duodenum, which is only about two feet in length, is strategically located near the stomach, pancreas, liver, and gallbladder. In addition to the stomach contents, it receives bile from the *liver* and *gallbladder* along with hormones and enzymes from the *pancreas* that assist with digestion. Dietary iron and calcium are predominantly absorbed into the body in the duodenum.

The *duodenum* is connected to the *jejunum* and *ileum,* which make up the remaining twenty or so feet of small intestine and are the site for the absorption of most nutrients. Hormones, with

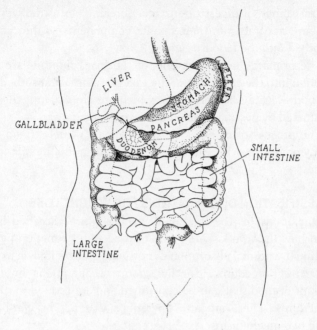

Figure 7-1: The GI Tract (2 views)

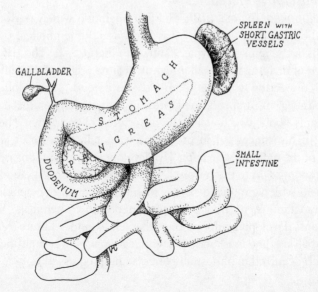

the assistance of digestive enzymes, break down carbohydrates, proteins, and fats into their smaller components so they can be absorbed into the bloodstream.

The primarily liquid contents of the *small intestine* are then emptied into the *colon*. Here, the excess water is reabsorbed into the body, leaving behind feces, which are stored until they are eliminated by passing through the *rectum* and *anus*.

The process of digestion is analogous to a finely tuned symphony orchestra, with each musician having a unique role in the process.

CLASSIFICATION OF OPERATIONS FOR WEIGHT LOSS

Operations for the treatment of obesity are classified based upon how they work. One group of procedures function by preventing the normal absorption of nutrients and are known as *malabsorptive* procedures. Another group of operations limit the amount of food that can be consumed and are termed *restrictive* procedures. There are also operations that act by combining these two mechanisms.

Malabsorptive Procedures

Jejunoileal Bypass (JIB): The first operation widely performed for the treatment of obesity was known as the jejunoileal bypass (JIB), or the intestinal bypass (shown in Figure 7-2). The JIB consisted of dividing the small intestine near its origin in the jejunum and connecting it to the ileum close to its end. This resulted in "bypassing" most of the small intestine (about eighteen feet), leaving only about two feet for the absorption of nutrients. The JIB was highly successful in producing weight loss; however, about half of the patients who had a JIB developed complications requiring readmission to the hospital. These adverse effects included diarrhea, which produced severe malnutrition and deficiencies in many vitamins, nutrients, and essential bodily chemicals. Some patients developed kidney stones that led to kidney failure, requiring dialysis. The most serious complication was liver malfunction, which occurred in almost all patients and progressed to fatal liver

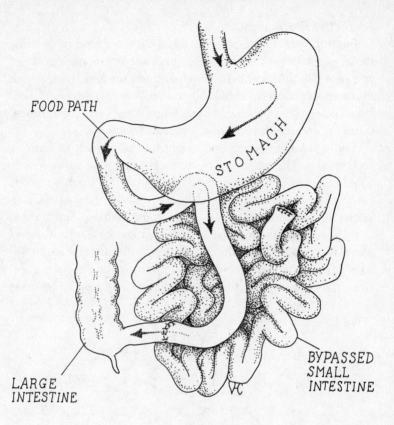

Figure 7-2: Jejunoileal Bypass (JIB)

failure in about 10 percent. This side effect could not be predicted, treated, or prevented.

The high incidence and severity of complications necessitated reversal of the procedure in about 25 percent of patients. For these reasons, JIB was abandoned by the surgical community in about 1980. It is currently the recommendation of the American Society for Bariatric Surgery that patients with an intact JIB undergo conversion to a safer weight loss procedure, even if they have no symptoms.

Restrictive Procedures

Gastroplasty: Gastroplasty is a general term used to describe those weight loss procedures that involve partitioning the stomach near the junction between the esophagus and the stomach into a small pouch that holds about one ounce. Because the partition is usually performed using surgical staplers, these procedures are commonly referred to "stomach staplings."

These procedures produce weight loss exclusively by limiting food intake. The gastroplasty works because one can eat only small amounts before becoming full. Eating too much stretches the pouch, causing pain, nausea, and vomiting. Numerous variations of gastroplasty were devised and subsequently abandoned because of a high rate of failure (Figure 7-3). Failure was often the result of technical problems related to the staples. Many times the staples pulled out, allowing the stomach to return to its normal size, thereby allowing food intake to increase

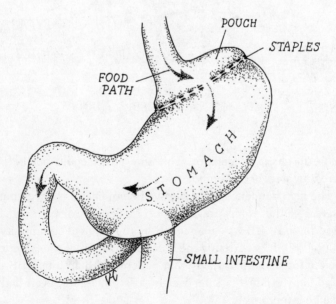

Figure 7-3: Gastroplasty

to pre-operative levels. The staplers currently in use are much improved and these problems are rare.

The form of gastroplasty in popular use today was introduced by Dr. Edward Mason in the 1970s and is known as vertical banded gastroplasty (VBG, Figure 7-4). This operation is performed by creating a one-ounce-size pouch near the junction of the stomach and esophagus, using a vertically placed staple line. The channel connecting the pouch to the remainder of the stomach is then reinforced with a permanent band (usually 1 cm [about ½ inch] in width and 5.5 cm [2½ inches] in length) made of silicone, Silastic, or polypropylene to prevent the opening from stretching. Food passes through the pouch into the rest of the stomach, where it is digested normally. The effectiveness of the operation is closely related to the size of the opening. Gastroplasty works by restriction only, by limiting the amount of food that can be eaten at one sitting. However, it can be

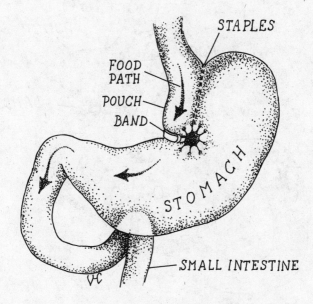

Figure 7-4: Vertical Banded Gastroplasty (VBG)

sabotaged by the ingestion of high-calorie, sweet liquids such as ice cream and shakes.

Gastric Banding: Gastric banding is a modification of gastro-plasty in which a stomach pouch is created by encircling the upper stomach with a Silastic or silicone band (Figure 7-5). This creates an hourglass appearance and functions by limiting the consumption of food and then delaying its passage into the rest of the stomach. Some of the bands are adjustable, allowing them to be loosened or tightened as needed. At this time, most of the clinical experience with gastric banding has been in Europe, Australia, and Israel. The laparoscopic adjustable gastric band was approved by the FDA for use in the United States in June 2001. Results in the U.S. have been mixed, with over a third of patients experiencing serious mechanical and technical problems, requiring removal or operative adjustment of the device.

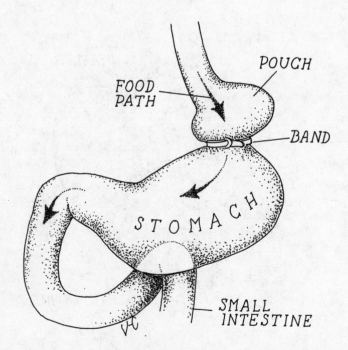

Figure 7-5: Gastric Banding

Combined Restrictive and Malabsorptive Procedures

Several procedures currently in use are a combination of restrictive and malabsorptive procedures.

Roux-en-Y Gastric Bypass (RYGB): The Roux-en-Y gastric bypass (Figure 7-6), which was also developed by Dr. Edward Mason, is the most popular bariatric procedure performed in the United States. It is a combination of restrictive and malabsorptive procedures. The restrictive component consists of making a small pouch near the junction of the esophagus and the stomach, using a surgical stapler. The malabsorptive portion is created by dividing the small intestine and rerouting it so that one portion is connected to the small stomach pouch (the *Roux limb* or *alimentary*

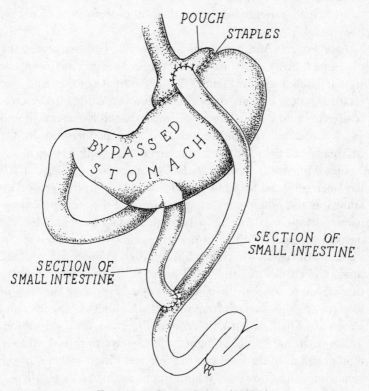

Figure 7-6: Gastric Bypass (RYGB)

limb) and the remaining portion, which delivers the bile and pancreatic juice, is reconnected to the small intestine at a predetermined distance from the stomach (the *bilio-pancreatic limb*).

Several variations of this procedure exist in which surgeons use different lengths for the alimentary and the bilio-pancreatic limbs. Lengths of the alimentary or bilio-pancreatic limb range from 30 cm (12 in.) to 250 cm (100 in.), with different surgeons using different combinations. Shorter limbs are referred to as *proximal* and longer limbs as *distal*. In patients who have a BMI less than 50, the limb length does not appear to affect the amount of weight loss. However, in heavier patients, with a BMI greater than 50, studies performed by Robert Brolin, M.D., and by Patricia Choban, M.D., and me have shown that longer alimentary-limb lengths—150 cm (60 in.) and 250 cm (100 in.)—helped patients lose more than 50 percent of their excess body weight.

Fobi Pouch: Another variant of the RYGB incorporates the placement of a band just before the connection between the stomach and jejunum (Figure 7-7). The purpose of the band is to retard the flow of food, as occurs with a vertical banded gastroplasty, and allow for a larger opening between the stomach and small intestine. This procedure has been popularized by Dr. Mathias A. L. Fobi and is often referred to as the *Fobi pouch*.

Bilio-Pancreatic Diversion (BPD): Since the 1980s, the JIB has been replaced by a more moderate malabsorptive procedure known as the bilio-pancreatic diversion or *Scopanaro procedure,* named after Dr. Nicola Scopanaro, the Italian surgeon who first devised it (Figure 7-8). This operation consists of several steps. First, about half of the stomach is removed in order to limit food intake. Then most of the small intestine is rerouted, similar to that which is done in the gastric bypass, to separate the flow of food leaving the stomach from the digestive juices of the liver and pancreas. This, in turn, decreases digestion and absorption. These paths are finally brought back together to mix as a "common channel" in the final two to three feet (50 to 100 cm) of the small intestine. However, malnutrition occurs in about 10 percent of patients, with additional nutritional deficiencies such as

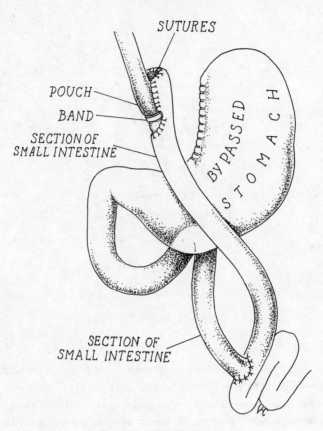

Figure 7-7: RYGB Variant

low calcium levels and bone disease in even more. This operation is popular in parts of Europe, especially Italy. Nevertheless, most bariatric surgeons in the United States feel that BPD is too radical an operation for most patients, and its precise role in the management of severe obesity remains to be determined. For these reasons, BPD was not evaluated during the NIH Consensus Development Conference on the Surgical Treatment of Obesity in 1991.

Bilio-Pancreatic Diversion with Duodenal Switch: A variation of the bilio-pancreatic bypass known as the *duodenal switch* (DS, Figure 7-9) has been developed in the United States by Douglas

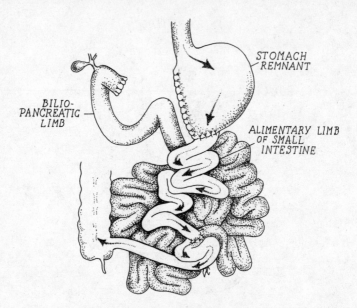

Figure 7-8: Bilio-Pancreatic Diversion (BPD)

Hess, M.D., and is currently preferred over the standard BPD by some surgeons in the United States and Canada. This modification involves connecting the rerouted small intestine to the duodenum instead of the stomach, which results in a lower incidence of stomach ulcers than the standard BPD. Only a few studies describing the long-term results of the DS have been published. The prevailing view of most bariatric surgeons in the United States is that DS, like BPD, is too radical for most patients, but that it probably has a limited role that remains to be determined.

Thus, of the "combined" procedures, the RYGB functions more like a restrictive procedure, while the BPD and the DS are more like malabsorptive procedures.

Note: The RYGB, BPD, and DS all involve division and reconstruction of the gastrointestinal tract using a technique called "Roux-en-Y," in which the intestine is reconnected in the shape of the letter Y. This technique was first employed by Cesar Roux, a

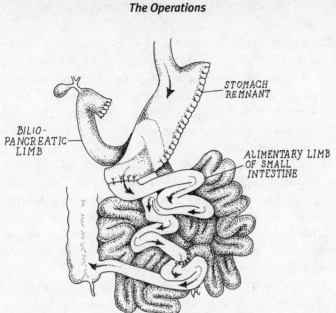

Figure 7-9: Duodenal Switch (DS)

Swiss surgeon in the late nineteenth century. The name credits him for the technique while describing the anatomy of the intestinal reconstruction. Thus, the abbreviation RNY, which is sometimes used for the Roux-en-Y gastric bypass, is inaccurate.

HOW DOES THE SURGERY WORK?

My surgeon explained to me how gastric bypass works. I'm not sure if I quite understand it all. All I know is that I can eat almost anything I enjoy, but I become full much faster. I eat much smaller portions, and consequently I've lost a lot of weight and kept it off for a long time.

Cathy T., 36, 327 lbs. pre-op; 189 lbs. 5 years post-op

I'm not even sure that doctors know exactly how this operation works—but the amazing part is that it does.

Jill M., 33, 306 lbs. pre-op; 173 lbs. 2 years post-op

The malabsorptive procedures produce weight loss by preventing the normal absorption of nutrients. The different procedures either short-circuit parts of the GI tract so that food passes through too quickly to be properly digested or absorbed, or they reroute the food so that it bypasses certain parts of the GI tract and does not come into contact with the hormones and juices necessary for digestion.

The restrictive procedures promote weight loss by limiting food intake through partitioning the stomach with staples or dividing it. When food enters this "smaller" stomach, the pouch quickly fills up, stretching the sides. Signals are then sent to the brain, indicating a feeling of fullness. If too much food is consumed and the pouch is stretched too quickly, pain followed by nausea and vomiting can result.

The combined procedures, which involve both restrictive and malabsorptive components, also appear to induce weight loss by altering the way the body uses energy. After a restrictive operation, patients consume small quantities of food for several months, usually about 500 calories per day after six weeks, 800 to 1,000 calories per day at six months, and 1,200 to 1,400 calories per day after one year. Such a low level of caloric intake is called semi-starvation. Normally, when people diet and consume such reduced amounts of food, the body interprets it as a threat to health. The body then compensates for this by lowering the amount of energy consumed in order to try to preserve body weight. Energy consumption can be reduced by as much as 30 percent, which is one of the primary reasons that it is often so difficult to lose weight by dieting alone. One purpose of combining exercise with dieting is to offset this reduction in energy utilization.

My colleague, Patricia Choban, M.D., and I measured the amount of energy expended by our patients who underwent RYGB. We found that despite the fact that they were consuming markedly reduced amounts of food than prior to surgery—between 500 and 1,200 calories per day, which should have caused a reduction in their energy use of 15 to 30 percent—their energy expenditure was normal. Earlier research involving patients who had a VBG, a purely restrictive operation, showed a reduction in energy consumption, similar to what happens when patients go on an ordinary diet. Thus, we believe that this "paradoxical response" after RYGB, in which patients maintain a normal level of energy use despite low caloric intake and do not demonstrate the expected slowdown in metabolic rate, may be responsible for the increased weight loss observed after RYGB when compared to VBG.

8

HOW SURGERY IMPROVES YOUR MEDICAL PROBLEMS

As a result of WLS, I'm not thin—but I'm not obese either. I can take a walk without huffing and puffing, and I can get down on the floor and play with my children.

MaryAnn W., 29, 274 lbs. pre-op; 149 lbs. 4 years post-op

My life has really changed because of my WLS. One of my biggest pleasures is now shoe shopping. Before the surgery, my feet were so swollen that I had to wear sneakers all the time. The other day, I bought a pair of high heels for the first time in ten years.

Tahisha K., 36, 344 lbs. pre-op; 217 lbs. 19 months post-op

Little things have changed, and that's what really makes a difference in my life. I don't have to ask for seat-belt extenders when I fly—and that's great.

Bill P., 44, 329 lbs. pre-op; 177 lbs. 5 years post-op

EFFECT OF WEIGHT LOSS SURGERY ON QUALITY OF LIFE

Surgical results should be analyzed from two perspectives. Traditionally, the medical profession has viewed the results of any therapy in terms of *efficacy*—how the specific problem or disease has been affected by the treatment. For example, how well did the treatment lower the blood sugar in people with diabetes or the blood pressure in patients with hypertension? The better the disease can be controlled or cured, the more effective the treatment. The same would hold true for weight loss.

However, during the past decade, emphasis has been given to analyzing the results of treatments from the patient's perspective. Medical science is beginning to examine how patients feel about the treatments they have undergone, separately from how a particular treatment affects the "numbers" (blood sugar, blood pressure, cholesterol level, etc.). This new focus on the *effectiveness* of medical treatments is referred to as "quality of life" or "medical-outcomes research," and it is particularly relevant to patients considering WLS. For example, we know that even modest amounts of weight loss (5 or 10 percent) can result in improvements in many obesity-related medical conditions, such as diabetes, high blood pressure, and high cholesterol. Imagine two individuals, both women who are 5 feet tall and weigh 300 pounds, with a BMI of 50. These women have diabetes, high blood pressure, and high cholesterol, and each takes the same medications. The first woman goes on an aggressive, medically supervised diet and loses 50 pounds in 6 months. After 1½ years, she has kept 40 pounds off. Although her final weight is 260 pounds, she is able to dispense with all of her medications. The second woman undergoes WLS and loses 140 pounds after 1½ years. Her weight is now 160 pounds and she too no longer takes any medications. Which woman do you think is happier with her result? If we analyzed this only from the perspective of efficacy, the treatments would be equivalent, because they had the same effect on the measured parameters—the levels of blood sugar, blood pressure, and cholesterol—and both resulted in elimination of the need for medications. However, if we factor in the effectiveness of the treatment on overall health and quality of life, the results would be quite different. The second woman is probably more satisfied from the patient's perspective, because she has lost an additional 120 pounds and can now shop in regular stores, sit in chairs without difficulty, and is more readily accepted by her coworkers. More and more, the results of medical treatments are being evaluated using quality-of-life indicators as well as traditional measures of efficacy, and this is also true in the analysis of the results of WLS.

EFFECT OF WEIGHT LOSS SURGERY ON MEDICAL PARAMETERS

I had to quit my job as a school-bus driver because I had such severe sleep apnea. After my surgery, that problem was cured. I got a better job—and life is looking good.

Tony S., 52, 523 lbs. pre-op; 316 lbs. 22 months post-op

Nobody understands why, but people who have gastric bypasses get the added bonus of having their diabetes cured. I went into the hospital taking insulin, and when I was discharged, I threw my insulin in the trash.

Lorraine G., 48, 286 lbs. pre-op; 154 lbs. 18 months post-op

My osteoarthritis wasn't cured after my WLS, but because I weighed so much less it eased some of the pressure on my joints. Surely, I'm not perfect, but I feel much better than I did before.

Stephanie V., 47, 311 lbs. pre-op; 214 lbs. 3½ years post-op

Weight Loss: Weight loss is the primary factor of concern to most patients considering WLS and the ultimate determinant of success. In the bariatric-surgery community, success has been defined as the loss of at least 50 percent of excess body weight. The weight is usually lost most rapidly during the first six months after surgery and then it begins to taper off and reaches a plateau after about one and a half to two years. In general, malabsorptive procedures result in the greatest weight loss, and restrictive procedures in the least.

The JIB (jejunoileal bypass), which is no longer performed, resulted in weight loss of approximately 80 percent of EBW. The BPD and DS (bilio-pancreatic diversion and duodenal switch) are almost as good in that regard, with weight losses approximating 70 to 80 percent of excess body weight. After RYGB (Roux-en-Y gastric bypass), patients typically lose between 50 and 75 percent of their excess body weight, while after VBG (vertical banded gastroplasty) they tend to lose between 40 and 60 percent of excess body weight. Early results of the adjustable lap banding procedures are comparable to VBG; however, most of the data comes from European studies in which the long-term follow-up has been poor. These results are summarized in Table 8-1.

Weight Regain: Data on weight regain parallel that on weight loss (Table 8-1). The malabsorptive procedures, JIB, BPD and DS, have the best results, with less than a 10 percent regain after 5 years and 10 years. RYGB is slightly less durable, with most studies reporting weight regain between 10 and 15 percent after 5 years, which continues as long as 15 years after surgery. VBG is less effective, with weight regain commonly as high as 25 to 40 percent after 5 years. Long-term data on gastric banding is not available as yet, but one can safely assume that it will be no better, and probably worse, than VBG.

Table 8-1: Weight Loss and Regain After Various Weight Loss Surgery Procedures

	JIB	BPD—DS	RYGB	VBG	Gastric Banding
Percent Excess Body Weight Lost	80	70–80	50–75	40–60	40–60
Percent Weight Regained	<10	<10	10–15	25–40	Unknown

POTENTIALLY LIFE-THREATENING CO-MORBID CONDITIONS

Weight loss by any means often results in considerable improvement or complete resolution of most obesity-related medical conditions. The degree of change is not necessarily related to the amount of weight loss. Improvement refers to a reduced requirement for treatment, whereas complete resolution implies cure, with no further treatment required.

Type II Diabetes: The effect of surgery (RYGB) on the course of type II diabetes is most dramatic. Studies by Dr. Walter Pories and colleagues from East Carolina University involving hundreds of patients have shown marked improvement in the biochemical abnormalities associated with diabetes. Within days of surgery, these investigators observed a return of fasting-blood-sugar levels to normal, lower blood levels of insulin (which are usually elevated because of the body's resistance to insulin), and most patients were able to be discharged from the hospital no longer needing insulin. The speed with which these improvements occurred suggests that they are not related to weight loss, since the amount of weight lost within the first few days of surgery is minimal.

Hypertension: Hypertension improves or completely resolves with weight loss in the vast majority of patients, with people taking lower doses of blood-pressure medication or no medication at all.

Hyperlipidemia: In most individuals, weight loss typically results in significant improvement in cholesterol and lipid abnormalities.

Cardiovascular Disease: Although long-term data on the risk of heart attack or stroke are not available, it seems reasonable to assume that elimination or reduction of predisposing factors for cardiovascular disease (diabetes, hypertension, lipid abnormalities) will reduce the overall cardiovascular risk.

Obstructive Sleep Apnea—Obesity Hypoventilation Syndrome (Pickwickian Syndrome): Marked improvement in sleep abnormalities after weight loss occurs in most people, with almost half experiencing complete resolution.

Liver Disease: Weight loss usually results in improvement in liver function and a decrease in fat deposits.

Cancer: It is unclear whether or not this risk decreases with weight loss.

The effect of surgery on several potentially life-threatening co-morbid conditions is summarized in Table 8-2.

Table 8-2: Effect of Weight Loss Surgery on Obesity-Related Co-morbid Conditions

Co-morbid Condition	Improved	Completely Resolved
Type II diabetes	93 percent	89 percent
Hypertension	90 percent	66 percent
Abnormal blood lipids	85 percent	70 percent
Sleep apnea	72 percent	40 percent

Lifestyle-Limiting Conditions

Weight loss also results in relief or improvement in most of these conditions, which often have a dramatic impact on people's lives.

Osteoarthritis: Weight loss relieves considerable strain on the lower back, hips, knees, and ankles. Patients often experience improved mobility and decreased requirements for anti-inflammatory or analgesic medications, allowing them to increase their activity level and productivity.

Gallstones: Rapid weight loss by any method is associated with an increased risk of gallstones. After WLS, this incidence is approximately 25 percent. In the past few years, a drug called ursodiol (Actigall, Urso250) has become available, which can reduce the risk to less than 5 percent.

Gastroesophageal Reflux: Heartburn usually resolves quickly with weight loss. In addition, regardless of its effect on weight, RYGB is an effective antireflux operation because it prevents the stomach acid from refluxing back into the esophagus.

Urinary Stress Incontinence: Symptoms of urinary stress incontinence are among the first to resolve with even modest degrees of weight loss.

Venous Disease: Mild symptoms of venous disease, such as varicose veins or transient leg swelling, can improve with weight loss. Unfortunately, patients with chronic venous disease or massive leg swelling often have permanent changes in their veins and skin by the time they are treated.

Menstrual Irregularity and Infertility: Ovulation, and hence menstrual periods, will often resume with weight loss. Consequently, many women who have had problems with infertility are able to conceive. There have been numerous reports of women having normal pregnancies after WLS, although it is recommended that birth control be used during the weight loss period.

Depression and Social Stigmatization: Numerous studies now document improvement in the symptoms of depression and low self-esteem after significant weight loss.

EFFECT OF WEIGHT LOSS SURGERY ON QUALITY-OF-LIFE MEASURES

I was missing so many days of work from obesity-related illnesses that I was terrified of losing my job. Now I only have to stay home when I have a cold.

Patrick O'C., 55, 366 lbs. pre-op; 204 lbs. 2½ years post-op

I have to buy a dress for my daughter's wedding and I'm not dreading it. When my son got married, I wore a size 26—now I fit nicely into a 16. I'm not a model, but I will make an attractive mother of the bride.

Sylvia F., 49, 286 lbs. pre-op; 193 lbs. 4 years post-op

Six months after my surgery I was able to fit comfortably behind the wheel of my car. That makes a tremendous difference in my life.

Barbara M., 34, 314 lbs. pre-op; 188 lbs. 20 months post-op

Information is accumulating concerning improvements in the quality of life of patients following WLS. Most of the results are positive. My colleague, Patricia Choban, M.D., and I published two of the first reports in the United States studying patients who underwent RYGB. Patients completed a standardized questionnaire called Short Form-36 (SF-36) before surgery and at different time points subsequently.

The SF-36 consists of thirty-six questions in eight categories: physical activity, social functioning, physical and emotional factors in role activities, bodily pain, general mental health, vitality, and general health perceptions, in which the patient grades his or her health in order to provide an assessment of overall health status. This questionnaire has been completed by thousands of patients nationwide and is widely used throughout the health-care system. Before surgery, patient responses were considerably below national norms in all of the areas assessed, indicating that their obesity severely compromised their health and limited their lives. Post-operatively, the patients showed a consistent improvement in their health status, to levels that either matched or exceeded the average.

These results reflect the positive effect that successful WLS has on patients' lives. Several studies in Europe have also documented marked improvement in quality of life, emotional well-being, and employment after WLS. These findings indicate that many of the psychological challenges confronted by severely overweight people are due to their weight, and not vice versa.

One of the more dramatic studies evaluating quality of life examined the negative effects of severe obesity compared to the positive effects of weight loss. Patients who had successful WLS were asked to compare their suffering from morbid obesity with several other conditions, such as diabetes, dyslexia, legal blindness, or having a leg amputated, combined with a normal weight. The patients overwhelmingly preferred to be normal weight with another disability than to be morbidly obese. When asked if they would accept several million dollars to remain morbidly obese, none chose the money over the opportunity to become normal weight.

Louis Martin, M.D., of Louisiana State University has documented that as many as 40 percent of patients who were receiving public assistance at the time of surgery were able to return to work after successful WLS. In Sweden, the Swedish Obesity Subjects (SOS) study is currently comparing the long-term effects of surgical and standard nonsurgical treatments in the largest prospective clinical trial of its kind in the world. Initial reports from the SOS have demonstrated the superiority of the surgical approach in all parameters, including medical outcomes and quality-of-life measures. The results of the SOS have also shown that surgery is cost effective; the operation pays for itself within three years as patients spend fewer health-care dollars on treatment of obesity-related medical problems and miss less time at work.

WLS is not magic or a panacea for all of life's problems. Researchers have documented that many patients will return to their baseline, pre-operative psychological profile several years after successful weight loss. These findings suggest that the psychological or social problems confronting obese individuals have multiple causes. Weight loss cannot improve an abusive marriage or make a "lousy" boss nicer.

However, examining all of the available information about WLS, balancing its risks, benefits, results, and costs, it is undeniable that it is the safest and most effective treatment for patients with clinically severe or morbid obesity.

9

CHOOSING THE RIGHT OPERATION

After much discussion with my friends on the Internet, I finally decided to approach my operation in a manner that I felt was logical. To the best of my ability, I selected a surgeon who I believed was experienced and well-qualified. I looked at his program and what it had to offer me in terms of follow-up care. Once I was satisfied that I had picked someone knowledgeable and caring, I decided to let him be in the driver's seat and pick which operation he thought was best for me. I'm an architect, and a very good one. I would really resent it if some surgeon tried to tell me how to design a building.

Walter L., 42, 456 lbs. pre-op; 311 lbs. 16 months post-op

THE PROCEDURE

Since most bariatric surgeons and patients had negative experiences with the intestinal-bypass or JIB, there has been a shift toward the use of more restrictive weight loss procedures. The desire to find safer operations led to the development of the vertical banded gastroplasty (VBG) and Roux-en-Y gastric bypass (RYGB) in the late 1960s and '70s. Initially, the VBG was more popular because it is simpler to perform and does not result in vitamin and mineral deficiencies. In the 1980s, approximately 75 percent of bariatric surgeons in the United States preferred the VBG, 25 percent preferred the RYGB, and less than 1 percent preferred more radical procedures like the bilio-pancreatic diversion or duodenal switch (BPD/DS).

However, over time it became apparent that VBG and other restrictive procedures are inferior to the RYGB in terms of weight loss achieved and weight regained. Thus, the pendulum has swung back toward more radical or malabsorptive weight loss procedures.

In a recent survey conducted by the American Society for Bariatric Surgery (1999), about 75 percent of surgeons preferred RYGB as their primary operation, 15 percent preferred VBG or a variation thereof, and 10 percent preferred BPD or DS. Comparing these three procedures (Table 9-1), the reasons for these preferences become clear. The VBG is the simplest procedure to perform; however, it results in less weight loss, more weight regain, and has the highest incidence of technical problems, which affect post-operative eating and often require re-operation.

The BPD/DS results in the greatest weight loss and smallest regain; however, it occasionally produces severe protein-calorie malnutrition, requiring reoperation and lengthening of the common channel. The RYGB results in good weight loss and maintenance, close to that achieved with BPD/DS, and does not cause the severe types of nutritional deficiencies (protein, calcium) that are occasionally seen after BPD/DS. Thus, most surgeons in the U.S. feel that, overall, RYGB is the best and safest operation available—with VBG being inferior and BPD/DS having too great a risk of complications.

With the development and perfection of newer procedures, surgical treatments for severe obesity should, logically, be more specifically tailored to the health risks and needs of individual patients. For example, VBG, gastric banding, and short-limb RYGB (less than 75 cm) may be best suited for individuals with the lowest BMIs (35 to 40 or 45); RYGB with longer limbs (150 to 250 cm) preferred for those with intermediate BMIs (40 or 45 to 55 or 60); and BPD/DS for those patients with the highest BMIs (over 55 or 60). Although intuitively this makes sense, carefully performed, long-term studies need to be done to document which operative procedures are best for which people.

Table 9-1: Comparison of Vertical Banded Gastroplasty, Roux-en-Y Gastric Bypass, Bilio-Pancreatic Diversion/Duodenal Switch

	VBG	RYGB	BPD/DS
Weight loss (percent of excess body weight lost)	40–60	60–75	70–80
Weight regain (percent of excess body weight regained)	25–40	10–15	<10
Limited amount of food intake	Yes	Yes	No
Types of food restricted	Meat, raw fruits and vegetables	Simple sugars and fats	Fats
Excessive gas/flatus	No	Rare	Common
Dumping syndrome*	No	Yes	No
Protein malnutrition	No	No	Occasional
Vitamin deficiency	No	Yes	Yes
Calcium deficiency	No	No	Yes
Iron, vit. B_{12} deficiency	No	Yes	Yes
Technical ease	Easiest	Intermediate	Most difficult
Need for operative revision	Common (weight regain, stricture, ulcer)	Rare (weight regain, stricture, ulcer)	Unusual (malnutrition, diarrhea)

* Dumping syndrome is a constellation of symptoms (light-headedness, cold sweats, abdominal cramps, and diarrhea) caused by certain foods, usually simple sugars or dense fats, leaving the stomach and entering the small intestine too quickly. It can occur after any operation that changes the way food is routed during digestion. (See Chapter 13 for more information about dumping syndrome and how to avoid it.)

THE METHOD: LAPAROSCOPIC OR OPEN

Until recently, all abdominal operations were performed through incisions that opened the abdomen, providing exposure to the internal structures. Laparoscopy is a method by which surgical procedures can be performed through a series of small incisions using specially made instruments and guided by a video camera. Although laparoscopy has been available for decades and has been widely used in gynecologic surgery for over twenty years, it only became popular in general surgery in the late 1980s, as a method to remove gallbladders (cholecystectomy). Since then, the equipment has improved considerably and laparoscopy has been increasingly used to perform other general surgery operations, including VBG, gastric banding, RYGB, and BPD/DS. Like all methods, laparoscopy has certain advantages and disadvantages. The major advantage of laparoscopy in WLS is related to the size of the incision. Rather than a formal incision in the midline, laparoscopy uses a series of five or six small incisions through which the camera and instruments are inserted. The disadvantages of laparoscopy include a considerably longer operating time, significant technical difficulties in performing the procedure that frequently lead to compromises in technique, and increased cost of equipment and personnel.

Based on experience with gallbladder surgery, the laparoscopic approach to WLS should result in less pain after surgery, fewer wound infections, fewer incisional hernias, shorter hospitalizations, and faster return to work. In fact, these advantages have only partly been realized. Post-operative pain is highly variable. The discomfort that patients experience spans a wide spectrum, with some having a great deal of pain and others having minimal pain. This is true of both the open and laparoscopic methods. Wound infections and incisional hernias (defects in the abdominal wall through which intestines or other parts can protrude) can and do occur after laparoscopy, although the incidence of hernias is lower than after open surgery. However, hernias in small incisions are more dangerous than hernias in large incisions, as the affected organs have a greater tendency to become trapped and die (develop gangrene). Even a low incidence of "strangulated" hernias after laparoscopy, which require emergency surgery to re-move portions of dead bowel that could possibly cause death, might be sufficient to offset any benefit of laparoscopy over open surgery.

The length of hospitalization with laparoscopic RYGB is usu-ally three to four days: Patients undergo surgery on the first day, begin liquids on the second day, and are discharged on the third day. In my practice of open RYGBs, I have replicated this routine and have been able to send the majority of my patients home on an identical schedule. Similarly, patients that do not have physi-cally demanding jobs can often return to work after one to two weeks, as they do after laparoscopy. It is unlikely that individuals with very physically demanding occupations will be back to work at full capacity much before four weeks with either technique.

On the other hand, several serious complications that usually require surgical treatment, such as leaks and internal hernias, oc-cur more frequently after laparoscopic than open surgery. In gen-eral, about 1 to 2 percent of patients having open VBG or RYGB report an incidence of leak. Early experience with the laparo-scopic technique has shown a leak rate as high as 4 percent. Internal hernias are hernias that occur within the abdomen when the intestine gets caught or twisted, causing a bowel obstruction. These hernias often result when the intestine is moved around during surgery and the openings created are not closed with stitches. With the open technique, it is routine to close these openings, thus preventing internal hernias from occurring. However, many surgeons performing laparoscopy do not routinely do so because it is technically challenging.

Some surgeons also make other modifications in gastric bypass technique when the procedure is done laparoscopically. For in-stance, they may alter the size of the anastomosis (opening be-tween the stomach and the intestine, through which food passes) and the route taken by the bowel. Only time and close follow-up will tell whether these changes affect the overall outcome and re-sults.

While a laparoscopic gastric banding takes about one hour to perform, laparoscopic VBG and RYGB take much longer to perform than open procedures. In the hands of an experienced surgeon, an open VBG or RYGB should take between forty-five and ninety minutes. BPD and DS are more complex procedures and require, on average, two to three hours. Laparoscopic procedures take considerably longer to accomplish than open procedures, with the operative time directly related to the skill and experience of the surgeon. A laparoscopic VBG takes between ninety minutes and three hours to perform, and a laparoscopic RYGB between two and six hours. At present, the shortest operative times with laparoscopy (when everything goes perfectly) seem to approximate the slowest times when done open (when complications are encountered). Numerous studies involving open surgery have documented that longer operative times are associated with a higher incidence of infectious complications. Whether this is true with laparoscopy is not yet known.

Laparoscopic procedures are also considerably more expensive. In addition to increased operating time, the costs are related to the video equipment required, the large number of expensive disposable staplers and laparoscopic instruments, and the need for an additional assistant in order to perform the procedure. In the case of gallbladder removal, where patients are usually discharged within twenty-four hours of surgery, the shorter length of hospitalization offsets the additional expenses in the operating room. However, if the length of stay is the same, then laparoscopy simply costs much more.

As is the case with all new technologies, laparoscopy must be carefully evaluated and compared to the existing standard treatment, which is the open technique. This is especially true in the area of WLS, where serious complications and poor results thirty years ago continue to tarnish this procedure's reputation and are responsible for much of the resistance and negativism patients and surgeons face within the lay and medical communities. Laparoscopic VBG and RYGB are new and the techniques being employed are constantly evolving. Technical changes in the performance of the operations are being made to make the procedure easier to perform through the laparoscope. Long-term follow-up is not yet available to compare the results of these modifications on weight loss or on the incidence of complications.

Recent data from the American Society for Bariatric Surgery shows that about two-thirds of bariatric operations are still done using open techniques and one-third are being done laparoscopically. This ratio is true for RYGBs, VBGs, and BPD/DS. Essentially all banding is done laparoscopically. Although laparoscopy is certainly here to stay, it is probably safe to say more studies are needed to better define which patients are the best candidates, which surgeons should be doing it, and what are the best techniques to perform.

10

COMPLICATIONS OF WEIGHT LOSS SURGERY

I had some complications after my WLS, but if I could go back in time, I would do it again in a minute.

Carly H., 46, 377 lbs. pre-op; 216 lbs. 5 years post-op

I was terrified of having serious complications during or after my WLS—that's why I put it off for so long. Looking back, I wish I had been braver—sooner.

Vicky D., 39, 319 lbs. pre-op; 192 lbs. 14 months post-op

I had a major complication following my operation. I had to stay in the hospital for an extra week. It was really scary for me and my family. But my surgeon was very reassuring. We got through it together, and now, two years later, I have no regrets.

Pam T., 58, 447 lbs. pre-op; 291 lbs. 2 years post-op

In the middle of the night my white count was elevated, and my body wasn't producing much urine. My surgeon was on the phone with the residents on and off for about an hour. At four A.M. he showed up in my room, looking pretty concerned. He thought that it was possible that I had a leak, and the only way he could find out for sure was to reoperate on me. "Bob," he said, "it's better to be safe than sorry." Off to the operating room I went, scared out of my wits. Luckily, he found the leak and repaired it, and I went home only a few days later than expected.

Bob C., 52, 477 lbs. pre-op; 307 lbs. 20 months post-op

Some complications result from the surgical procedure itself, while others are the result of the nutritional alterations caused by the operation.

COMPLICATIONS DUE TO THE SURGICAL PROCEDURE

All operations are associated with complications and risks, and all surgeons have patients who experience them. Fortunately, the incidence of complications is low. Some complications are general and can occur after any type of surgery, while others are more closely related to the specific type of operation performed. The occurrence of a complication does not automatically imply that the patient or the surgeon did anything wrong.

The risks of WLS are higher than other types of gastrointestinal surgery because the patients are already at greater risk than their normal-weight counterparts.

All of the people who undergo WLS have severe obesity, and, as we discussed earlier, merely having clinically severe obesity predisposes one to early death in addition to all of the associated medical problems. Because there are no normal-weight individuals undergoing WLS, it stands to reason that the risks associated with WLS will be higher than those reported for many standard abdominal operations, which are performed on both normal-weight and overweight people. In fact, the risks that we will discuss actually apply to all people with severe obesity undergoing any major operative procedure under general anesthesia.

Possible Surgical Complications of WLS

Death: Death can occur as a result of any surgical procedure. The risk of death in several large studies of patients undergoing WLS is about 1 percent, or one out of 100 patients. However, the risk may vary from patient to patient depending upon the individual's associated medical problems and overall health. It may be as low as 0.5 percent (one in 200 patients) or as high as 4 percent (one in 25 patients). It is impossible to predict which patients will die in any given case. However, clinically severe obesity is a serious and life-threatening problem, and many patients have associated medical problems that increase this risk, such as sleep apnea, hypertension, coronary artery disease, and diabetes. In my opinion, the patients who are sickest as a result of their obesity are those that most need the surgery, since there are no other effective treatments to offer them. However, this group also has the greatest number of complications and the highest risk of death.

Cardiac Problems: Cardiac problems can occur after any operation but are more common in patients who already have angina, heart failure, hypertension, high cholesterol, and diabetes. Myocardial infarction (heart attack) is extremely rare. I have seen only one in caring for over 1,200 gastric-bypass patients. A more common problem in this population is sudden cardiac death, which is caused by a sudden change in the rhythm of the heart (arrhythmia). Severely obese patients are at increased risk for sudden cardiac death at a rate about eight times greater than normal-weight individuals. This may not be a preventable complication, although some patients show irregularities on their pre-operative electrocardiogram (ECG) and can be monitored.

Pulmonary Complications: Patients undergoing abdominal operations under general anesthesia typically experience the collapse of small portions of their lungs. This collapse is termed *atelectasis* and usually manifests itself as a fever on the night of surgery. This complication usually resolves with simple maneuvers such as early walking (which is why we encourage patients to get out of bed and walk as soon as possible after surgery), coughing and deep-breathing exercises, and chest physiotherapy. Untreated atelectasis can progress to pneumonia if the collapsed portions do not reexpand. Pneumonia is a more serious complication, requiring treatment with antibiotics, which can often prolong hospitalization and delay recovery. Although it is commonly believed that obese patients are at markedly greater risk for the development of post-operative pneumonia, a careful review of the medical literature and my own clinical experience indicate that the incidence of pneumonia is very low if the operation is completed in a reasonable length of time (under ninety minutes) and appropriate precautions are aggressively instituted.

Blood Clots: The formation of blood clots in the large veins of the legs and within the pelvis (deep vein thrombosis) is a serious problem because portions of these clots can break off and travel to the lungs (pulmonary embolism), causing death. Obese patients are at increased risk for the development of blood clots and, therefore, precautions should be taken before, during, and after surgery. Low doses of heparin (a blood thinner) can be administered, and pneumatic-compression stockings (which are devices similar to blood-pressure cuffs that are applied to the legs and stimulate blood flow by continually inflating and deflating) may be used. These measures, either alone or together, should be initiated before surgery for optimal effect and continued until the patient is fully ambulatory. It is not known if the combination is better than either treatment alone.

The incidence of deep vein thrombosis is less than 5 percent. Signs and symptoms suggestive of deep vein thrombosis, such as leg swelling and pain, are not specific and may be associated with many other ailments. Hence, many patients go undiagnosed unless the more serious complication of a pulmonary embolism occurs. Patients with a pulmonary embolism are usually short of breath, have a rapid heart rate, and may complain of chest pain. These manifestations are also not specific and can occur with many conditions, such as pneumonia or a heart attack. However, such symptoms or signs suggest a potentially serious problem and that a diagnostic work-up is indicated. Tests usually include a chest X ray, electrocardiogram (ECG), and a measurement of the oxygen level in the blood. Other tests may be indicated depending on the results.

If the diagnosis of a deep vein thrombosis or pulmonary embolism is confirmed, blood thinners are administered (anticoagulation). Usually, heparin is initially given by vein and then switched to a drug called Coumadin, which is taken orally. Anticoagulation drugs are usually continued for about six months.

Leak: A leak happens when one of the sutures or staple lines closing off the intestine or between two parts of the intestine that have been sewn together does not hold. This allows the digestive juices that are normally inside the intestine to leak into the abdominal cavity, where they can cause a severe infection, similar to those that occur with a perforated ulcer or a ruptured appendix. Leaks can complicate any intestinal operation and are not more common following WLS. The incidence of leaks in patients having their first operation for weight loss is about 1 percent. In patients undergoing a second operation, such as conversion of a failed VBG to an RYGB, the risk is higher, about 4 percent, because of the adhesions (scarring) in the area that make the operation more difficult.

The only way to prevent leaks is by employing safe surgical techniques. Most surgeons check for leaks during the operation by injecting air or colored solution into the stomach and seeing if anything "leaks" out. However, this is not foolproof and only checks for openings in the suture and staple lines in the stomach. Because their appearance may be delayed, many surgeons also test for leaks post-operatively before initiating feedings with an upper-GI study, in which gastrograffin (a liquid similar to barium that can be seen on an X ray) is swallowed and X-ray pictures taken.

Leaks are a serious complication and usually require an operation to identify the site of the leak and repair it. Often, if a leak is identified quickly, it is easily repaired and prolongs the hospitalization and recovery by only a few days. However, sometimes the infection within the abdomen can be severe and the repair difficult. In these cases, the patient may require treatment in the intensive-care unit followed by a lengthy hospitalization and recovery. Infrequently, deaths can occur as the result of leaks.

In my experience, most leaks are detected clinically on the first or second day after surgery. Patients simply do not look or feel well and often seem disoriented. They may or may not complain of abdominal pain. Patients may be short of breath, have a rapid heart rate, low urine output, and an elevated white-blood-cell count. The diagnosis can be confirmed with X-ray studies (a gastrograffin UGI or CAT scan). However, in my experience, the most prudent course of action when a leak is suspected is to re-operate as quickly as possible. A fast response is the surest way to confirm the diagnosis and repair the damage early. The effects of a negative exploratory laparotomy, where no leaks are discovered, are minimal compared to the benefits of fixing the leak sooner.

Occasionally, a leak may present "late," as an abscess. In these cases it can often be treated by placement of a drain, avoiding another operation.

Injury to the Spleen: The spleen is a fragile organ that is situated in the left upper portion of the abdomen, adjacent to the stomach. In about 1 percent of cases, it is accidentally injured during stomach operations. Most of the time it can be repaired; however, sometimes it cannot and must be removed. This may add about thirty minutes to the procedure and in rare cases requires a blood transfusion.

The consequences of removing the spleen (splenectomy) in an adult are minimal. This organ participates in the immune system by helping recognize and filter certain bacteria. However, by the time people are adults, they have already been exposed to most of these germs so that the antibodies have already been made.

Marginal Ulcer: In RYGB and BPD, a portion of the small intestine is sewn to the stomach. This connection between the stomach and small intestine is not normal, and the small intestine is therefore prone to develop ulcers, called *marginal ulcers,* from the strong acid contained in the stomach. Aspirin and nonsteroidal antiinflammatory drugs (NSAIDs), such as ibuprofen, can also cause these ulcers.

Patients with ulcers usually complain of pain, but they can experience excessive nausea and vomiting. In some cases, the ulcer can bleed, which results in either vomiting blood or passing black or maroon-colored stool. The diagnosis of an ulcer is most often made by upper-GI endoscopy, a procedure in which a scope is passed into the stomach so the stomach and intestine can be examined. The incidence of marginal ulcers in my practice is about 1 percent.

Most of these ulcers can be treated successfully with anti-ulcer medications called H_2-blockers (such as Tagamet, Zantac, and Pepcid) or proton pump inhibitors (Prilosec, Prevacid, Nexium). The usual course of drug treatment is eight to twelve weeks, at which time the endoscopy should be repeated. In the rare instance that an ulcer is resistant to drug therapy, surgery may be necessary.

Stricture: Strictures are narrowings that block the passage of food going down the GI tract. They are usually the result of excessive scarring and most commonly occur after a VBG at the site of the band in the stomach. Strictures occur less frequently after RYBG, where the stomach and small intestine are sewn together.

Patients with strictures usually complain of prolonged difficulty tolerating solids or liquids and excessive vomiting. The diagnosis can be confirmed with a UGI X ray or endoscopy. Treatment can often be accomplished by endoscopy, where a balloon attached to the outside of the scope is passed into the stricture and inflated under pressure to dilate the narrow channel and reopen the passageway. This is similar to the procedure of angioplasty that is performed on the heart. Unfortunately, after balloon dilation, the scarring usually recurs and surgery is eventually necessary. In the case of a VBG, the recommended operation is conversion to an RYGB. The incidence of strictures in my practice is about 2 percent.

Wound Infection: Obese patients have thick abdominal walls and are therefore prone to develop wound infections. The incidence of wound infections in obese patients after abdominal surgery can be as high as 10 percent, compared to a rate of 2 percent in normal-weight patients. Although wound infections are not life-threatening, their treatment is often time-consuming and can significantly delay recovery and return to work. Wound infections also increase the tendency to develop hernias in the incision.

Prevention of all wound infections, while theoretically possible, is not feasible. However, some precautions can be taken. All patients undergoing WLS should receive prophylactic (preventive) antibiotics, which are administered before surgery and continued for the day of the operation. I have been able to reduce the rate of wound infections in my patients to about 2 percent by leaving a drain in the subcutaneous fat to suck out the fluid that accumulates in the wound. In addition, I close the skin with a continuous "plastic surgery" stitch, which does not require removal and is more cosmetically appealing. The incidence of wound infections after laparoscopy also appears to be in the range of 2 percent.

Incisional Hernia: An incisional hernia is caused by a defect in the abdominal wall through which fat or intestine within the abdomen protrudes. Patients may have no symptoms or experience a variety of complaints, including pain, vomiting, diarrhea, or constipation. In the worst circumstance, a portion of intestine can become entrapped in the hernia site, requiring an emergency operation.

Incisional hernias occur in less than 5 percent of patients in my practice but have been reported in up to 20 percent of patients after obesity surgery performed by the open method. The incidence is lower when done laparoscopically (see Chapter 9 for more on this issue). A huge amount of tension is placed upon the stitches holding the abdomen closed in severely obese patients, and in a small percentage of cases, either the tissue or the stitches do not hold. Most incisional hernias will slowly continue to enlarge over time and will ultimately require surgery. In general, it is best to delay repair until most of the weight has been lost, which will make the repair easier and increase the chance for success. Most incisional hernias can be fixed by resuturing the tissues. However, in the case of larger hernias, an artificial material (mesh) may be necessary to close or reinforce the defect. It is sometimes possible to have a large abdominal pannus removed (abdominoplasty, or "tummy tuck") at the same time.

Intestinal Obstruction: An intestinal or bowel obstruction is a blockage that prevents food and liquid from progressing through the intestine. A bowel obstruction can result in infection, perforation, or death if not detected and treated early. If the blockage is partial, it can often resolve without surgery; however, complete obstructions almost invariably require an emergency operation to correct. Any patient who undergoes an abdominal operation is at a 1 percent risk for an intestinal or bowel obstruction.

The most common cause of post-operative bowel obstructions are adhesions, which are bands of scar tissue that form between different parts of the intestine or between the intestine and other structures. At surgery, these bands can be cut to free the bowel and relieve the blockage. If the blood supply to the intestine has been compromised, removal of a segment of intestine is necessary.

Another, less common type of intestinal obstruction is an internal hernia. An internal hernia occurs when a piece of intestine becomes trapped within an opening in the abdomen, causing a blockage. This complication often occurs when openings within the abdomen to reroute parts of the intestine have been made and not closed, thus allowing the bowel to slip through the opening and become caught. Internal hernias are especially dangerous because they frequently result in compromises to the intestinal blood supply and require removal of a gangrenous portion of intestine.

Although both of these types of obstructions are relatively uncommon after WLS, they can occur. Adhesive bowel obstructions are probably more common after open surgery, whereas internal hernias are more common after the laparoscopic approach.

NONSURGICAL COMPLICATIONS CAUSED BY THE PROCEDURE

Protein-Calorie Malnutrition: Malabsorptive procedures produce significant malabsorption of nutrients more frequently than the restrictive procedures. The highest incidence occurs after JIB (20 to 60 percent), followed by BPD and DS (2 to 10 percent). The incidence of clinically significant malnutrition is essentially zero after RYGB and VBG and is probably not an issue after gastric banding, although that information is unavailable. These results are shown in Table 10-1.

Micronutrient and Vitamin Deficiency: Malabsorption of micronutrients, such as iron and calcium, and vitamins, especially B_{12} and folic acid, is more common than protein-calorie malnutrition. All of the procedures that have a malabsorptive component (such as RYGB, BPD, and DS) and bypass the lower stomach and duodenum can cause micronutrient and vitamin deficiencies (see Table 10-1). For this reason, surgeons routinely prescribe vitamins and monitor blood levels of iron, vitamin B_{12}, and calcium after surgery.

Diarrhea: Malabsorption is frequently associated with diarrhea. After JIB, virtually 100 percent of patients experienced diarrhea. This side effect necessitated readmitting about 25 percent of patients to the hospital. BPD and DS are occasionally complicated by diarrhea, and many of these patients produce foul-smelling stool because of the malabsorption of fat. Diarrhea is rare after RYGB and VBG, with some patients even complaining of constipation. I believe that difficulty having bowel movements is due to patients not consuming enough liquids post-operatively.

Table 10-1: Metabolic Complications after Various Weight Loss Surgery Procedures

	JIB	BPD/DS	RYGB	VBG	Gastric Banding
Protein-Calorie Malnutrition	20–60 percent	2–10 percent	0	0	0
Micronutrient & Vitamin Deficiency	40–90 percent	30–50 percent	10–20 percent	<5 percent	<5 percent
Diarrhea	100 percent	10 percent	<5 percent	0	0
Dumping Syndrome	0	0	50–100 percent	0	0
Electrolyte Abnormalities	70–100 percent	<5 percent	0	0	0

Electrolyte Abnormalities: Serum electrolytes are chemicals such as sodium, potassium, chloride, and magnesium. These elements are some of the necessary components of cells and are required for normal heart function and many chemical reactions in the body. Electrolyte abnormalities can occur when large amounts of fluid are lost through vomiting, diarrhea, and after excess urine output (which can occur from taking water pills). This imbalance occurred frequently after JIB, often necessitating readmission to the hospital, and it occurs much less frequently after BPD and DS. Electrolyte imbalances are extremely rare following RYGB, VBG, or gastric banding.

Hair Loss: Hair loss (alopecia) can occur with any form of stringent dieting and weight loss, or due to a variety of causes (Table 10-2). After WLS, approximately 10 to 20 percent of patients experience hair that is thinning or easily removed during routine combing or brushing. Protein and iron deficiencies are probably the most common causes of hair loss after WLS. These are best treated by increasing the amount of protein consumed in the diet and by taking iron supplements (which require a prescription). If it is going to occur, hair will start thinning about three to six months after surgery and will usually stop falling out after six to nine months, after which time the hair will grow back. Most protein malnutrition occurs immediately after surgery, when patients are least able to ingest an adequate amount of protein. It takes three months for the effects to become evident in the body. Thus, loss of hair represents protein malnutrition that

Table 10-2: Causes of Hair Loss after Weight Loss Surgery:

Several factors, alone or in combination, can contribute to hair loss.

Insufficient protein and calorie intake

Iron deficiency

Vitamin and trace-element deficiencies

Major systemic stress (e.g., surgery, high fevers, psychological trauma)

Liver and other chronic systemic diseases (e.g., lupus, inflammatory bowel disease)

Drugs

ACE inhibitors (e.g., captopril, enalapril)—taken for high blood pressure

Allopurinol—taken for gout

Anticoagulants (e.g., Coumadin)—taken for blood clots

Antidepressants—taken to treat depression

Antithyroid medications

β-blockers (e.g., propanolol, atenolol)—taken for heart disease and high blood pressure

Birth-control pills

Cimetidine (Tagamet)—taken to reduce stomach acid

Lithium—taken for manic-depressive disorder

Ursodiol (Actigall, Urso250)—taken to prevent gallstones

occurred three months earlier; therefore, taking in extra protein at the actual time of hair loss is ineffective. Eating as much protein as possible right after surgery, including the use of protein shakes and supplements, is helpful. If you are taking any medications that can cause hair loss, consult your physician so that an alternative treatment can be prescribed. DO NOT stop any prescription medication on your own.

Excessive Gas: Patients occasionally complain of excessive gas after gastric-bypass surgery. In the most troublesome cases, this

Table 10-3: Foods Associated with Excess Gas Formation:

Highly gaseous foods:

milk, milk products, onions, beans, celery, prunes, Brussels sprouts, cauliflower, broccoli, tomatoes, asparagus, carrots, raisins, bananas, apricots, pretzels, bagels, wheat germ

Moderately gaseous foods:

pastries, eggplant, potatoes, lettuce, cucumber, peppers, avocado, zucchini, okra, olives, citrus fruit, apples, bread

Table 10-4: Remedies for Excess Gas:

For individuals with lactose intolerance or deficiency, many lactose-free milk products are commercially available. Alternatively, preparations of lactase are available (Lactaid drops, Lactaid caplets, and Lactrase capsules) that can be added to regular milk products in order to assist in their digestion.

For individuals with intolerance to legumes and vegetables, a new enzyme product (Beano) is available that can be used to help with digestion and may be effective in controlling the gas. Five to eight drops are placed on the food before eating. Food should not be hot, because the heat will inactivate the enzyme.

Avoid sugar-free foods made with sugar substitutes such as sorbitol and fructose.

Oral bismuth products (e.g., Pepto-Bismol), activated charcoal (Charcoal Plus, Flatulex, Charcocaps), and antacids (Mylanta, Maalox, Riopan) may decrease the effects of the bacteria or absorb intestinal gas.

takes the form of frequent and foul-smelling flatus, which can be embarrassing in public.

The excessive gas is usually related to dietary factors. After gastric bypass, certain foods are not digested normally by the time they reach the large intestine or colon, where the gas is formed and then excreted. The most common of these foods are: dairy or milk products containing lactose if the individual is lactose-deficient; certain legumes or vegetables, because humans do not have enzymes necessary for their digestion; and certain sugar substitutes, such as sorbitol and fructose, which are also incompletely digested. The following tables contain a list of foods that can cause excess gas after WLS (Table 10-3) and remedies (Table 10-4).

OTHER CONSIDERATIONS

Length of Surgery: The length of the operative procedure is significant for several reasons. Many studies have documented an increase in the incidence of infectious complications, such as pneumonia and wound infection, after prolonged open surgical procedures. These complications may be related to the fact that longer procedures result in a fall in body temperature, which in turn interferes with the immune system. Furthermore, longer operative times mean increased exposure to general anesthesia, which often results in the collapse of portions of the lung and can lead to pneumonia. In general, shorter operations are safer.

Longer operations are also more expensive. The cost of running an operating room is quite high, with expensive equipment and highly trained personnel. In addition, complications due to prolonged surgery result in longer hospital stays and increase costs.

Length of Hospital Stay: Although people go to hospitals in order to get well, staying in hospitals is unhealthy. Longer hospital stays expose patients to dangerous bacteria and viruses that live in hospitals, and therefore there is a greater chance they will acquire an infection. This risk is even greater after an individual undergoes surgery, which is an invasive procedure. Consequently, the shorter the stay, the better.

Because cost is closely related to the length of the stay, most hospitals try to discharge people as early as possible. Obviously, there needs to be a balance between sending patients home too early, which can result in complications and readmission to the hospital, and allowing them to stay too long.

AVOIDING COMPLICATIONS

Of course, many complications are beyond your control, but there are some basic steps that everyone can take to minimize the chances of developing them or to prevent them from becoming serious:

Call your doctor when you experience symptoms that alarm you. Don't try to be stoic and tell yourself that they will go away. Your doctor can only help you if (s)he knows what's happening to you. Some symptoms may warrant immediate medical attention, such as the sudden onset of severe chest or abdominal pain or shortness of breath. The key factors in determining whether a problem is serious enough to arouse concern are the suddenness and severity of the symptom.

Follow your doctor's instructions, especially with respect to medications and diet. You have taken a serious step to improve your health and don't want to undermine it by taking unnecessary risks.

Begin exercising as soon as feasible. Walking is best at first, as soon as possible, even if it hurts some. Walking improves your breathing and decreases your chances of developing pneumonia and blood clots.

Use the little breathing machine they give you in the hospital. It will exercise your lungs and decrease the chance of developing pneumonia.

REVISIONS

Gail B., 49, 344 lbs. pre-revision; 236 lbs. 1 year post-revision

I had my first WLS in 1989—a vertical banded gastroplasty. My surgeon was an older man who was a kind of pioneer in the field. When I went in for the operation I was 350 pounds, and within a year I weighed 230. I tolerated liquids well, but when I attempted solids, I usually vomited. Certain foods, like fruits, vegetables, and meat, were particularly difficult for me to digest. Losing the weight was wonderful, but spending hours each week with my head in the toilet bowl was terribly unpleasant.

In order to fend off nausea, my diet was restricted to things like milk shakes, soda, and mashed potatoes. Since I couldn't eat a healthy, well-balanced diet, my weight began creeping back up. Nine years postoperatively, I was 47 years old and 344 pounds— within a few pounds of my pre-operative weight.

Discouraged does not even begin to describe how I felt. My surgeon had retired, so I had no one to turn to for guidance. I couldn't help but wonder if WLS had been a terrible idea from the get-go. I decided to make an appointment with my internist to discuss my concerns. He told me that WLS was out of his realm of expertise. But he did give me a good piece of advice; he recommended a hospital known for the treatment of obesity. "Why don't you go there and see what they have to say?"

Feeling as if I didn't have much of a choice, I called the hospital for an appointment with an obesity specialist, who then referred me to a surgeon. I wasn't sure if this was the route I wanted to take again, but I figured I should hear what he had to say. Arriving in his office, I felt immediately reassured after hearing how many people were in my situation after a VBG. Somehow, I thought that I was atypical and what had happened to me was my fault. The surgeon explained that this was a common problem after the VBG and that it was not my fault. He told me that many surgeons had switched to doing the gastric bypass over the VBG because of these problems. Then he showed me how he could convert the VBG to a gastric bypass. He told me that after it was all over, I would lose weight and be able to eat a wider variety of foods than before—just in much smaller portions. I told him that I had some things to think about and I went home to figure this all out.

Impulsively, I picked up the phone and called information and got the phone number of the man who had done my VBG. I apologized profusely for calling him at home. He was most gracious and told me that, at the time, VBG was a state-of-the-art operation. However, from what he had read, gastric bypass was a huge improvement.

Some decisions are partially a leap of faith—but I have a lot of faith that things happen for a reason. I called and made an appointment for surgery. The insurance approval was a little tricky because I had already failed one procedure, but the surgeon and my internist wrote strong letters of medical necessity. I remembered the ropes—not eating after midnight the night before, and the pain I would feel afterward. I was prepared for that if I could just get back to a more normal weight. I also knew that painkillers had improved since my last foray into the operating room and that I could even control the dosage of medication myself.

Revisions can be much more complicated than gastric bypasses and they take longer to complete. I was in the operating room for about two hours. The surgeon said that it was a technically difficult operation because I had a lot of scar tissue between my liver and my stomach from the VBG. However, I came through it well. I started a soft diet on the second day after surgery and went home on the fourth.

It's been a year now since my revision. I've lost 108 pounds and I'm eating foods that I hadn't touched in years. Last night for dinner I had a small piece of lean meat, some broccoli, and a salad. I'm thrilled to be able to go out to a restaurant with my family and not have my food through a straw. Converting from VBG to gastric bypass was one of the biggest decisions of my life—and also one of the best.

Revisions of previous weight loss procedures are done for several reasons:

Technical complications, such as strictures or nonhealing ulcers;

Metabolic complications, such as malnutrition, severe diarrhea, or vitamin and mineral deficiency;

Weight regain;

Insufficient weight loss.

Reoperative surgery is more complicated than primary surgery. Intellectually, the surgeon must understand precisely what was done at the original operation and determine the nature of the current problem in order to formulate an appropriate corrective plan. This usually requires obtaining a copy of the operative report and may require X-ray studies, such as an upper-GI series, CT scan, or an endoscopy. Technically, revisions are more demanding because scarring and adhesions in the area make the identification and dissection of the tissues harder and increase the potential for injury to the main structures involved and to adjacent organs. For example, in the course of a revision of a VBG, the surgeon may encounter adhesions of the stomach and small intestine to the abdominal wall, adhesions of the liver to the stomach, and adhesions of the spleen to the stomach. The act of freeing up the stomach pouch to begin the corrective procedure could lead to extensive bleeding from the liver or spleen or injury to the stomach or intestine, requiring blood transfusion, removal of the spleen, or removal of a portion of the stomach or intestine. Because revisions are more challenging, they usually take longer than primary cases and are associated with a higher incidence of complications. A reasonable estimate is that the time and risk of complications is one and a half to two times as great. In my practice, most primary gastric bypass procedures take about an hour and most revisions between one and a half to two hours. I always leave a nasogastric tube in place after a revision and wait an extra day before beginning to feed patients. In addition, the incidence of leaks with revisions is about 2 percent and the need for a splenectomy is about 2 percent. The length of hospitalization may also be prolonged by several days after a revision.

The type of operation performed is dependent on the previous procedure and the problem being corrected. For example, most complications of a VBG, such as persistent vomiting due to a stricture, pain due to a nonhealing ulcer, or weight regain because of a high-caloric diet or staple-line disruption, can be corrected by converting the VBG to an RYGB. Similar technical complications after RYGB, on the other hand, must be managed without taking apart the gastric bypass, which can be more difficult. Insufficient weight loss or weight regain after RYGB is usually handled by lengthening the bypass (shortening the common channel). When this is done, care must be taken to avoid creating too short a common channel, which can lead to diarrhea, vitamin and mineral deficiency, and malnutrition. Revisions after BPD/DS are most commonly the result of diarrhea, vitamin and mineral deficiency, or malnutrition, and are managed by lengthening the common channel, thus providing more length for the absorption of nutrients. JIBs can be converted to a VBG, RYGB, or BPD/DS. (These are summarized in Table 10-5.)

Table 10-5: General Scheme for Revisions of Weight Loss Operations

Original Operation	Complication	Corrective Procedure
Vertical Banded Gastroplasty (VBG)	Stricture Nonhealing ulcer Staple-line disruption Weight regain Inadequate weight loss	Convert to RYGB
Roux-en-Y Gastric Bypass (RYGB)	Stricture Nonhealing ulcer Weight regain Inadequate weight loss	Revise connection between stomach and small intestine Lengthen bypass (shorten common channel)
Bilio-Pancreatic Diversion (BPD)	Nonhealing ulcer	Convert to DS
Bilio-Pancreatic Diversion with Duodenal Switch (BPD/DS)	Malnutrition Severe vitamin/ mineral deficiency Severe diarrhea	Shorten bypass (lengthen common channel)
Jejunoileal Bypass (JIB)	Malnutrition Severe vitamin/ mineral deficiency Severe diarrhea	Convert to VBG, RYGB, or BPD/DS

REVERSALS OF WLS PROCEDURES

Any weight loss procedure should be thought of as a permanent solution, because if it is reversed, the weight will be regained. Although technically feasible, reoperative surgery is much more difficult and complex and the result will NOT, in all likelihood, restore the individual to their exact same state as before surgery. This can be thought of as similar to remodeling a house. If you knock down walls and add rooms and floors, it's usually permanent. Although they can be knocked down again and rebuilt, such a procedure would typically be very complicated and expensive, and the result not necessarily identical to the original.

11

THE SURGERY: WHAT TO EXPECT BEFORE, DURING, AND AFTER

One definition of major surgery is *any surgery performed on me.* WLS is major surgery by any criteria. For this reason, it is perfectly reasonable for anyone contemplating WLS to ask questions about and be familiar with what to expect before, during, and after the operation.

WHAT TO EXPECT BEFORE SURGERY (PRE-OPERATIVELY)

I was a nervous wreck the night before my surgery. I couldn't sleep a wink. Like most people, I'm afraid of the unknown.

Robert R., 43, 689 lbs. pre-op; 425 lbs. 1 year post-op

I was glad that one of my friends from the Internet told me to bring a book with me. Reading really distracted me while I was waiting for the surgery to start.

Maureen G., 49, 485 lbs. pre-op; 321 lbs. 14 months post-op

My surgeon recommended that I meet with the anesthesiologist the week before the operation. Talking to him allayed many of my deepest fears about being put to sleep.

Elizabeth L., 58, 375 lbs. pre-op; 244 lbs. 3½ years post-op

The First Steps

Surgical Consultation: The first step in having WLS is an initial consultation with a surgeon. (Tips for helping you select a surgeon are discussed in a separate chapter.) At the first visit, the surgeon should obtain a thorough health history, including information about your weight, previous attempts at weight loss, associated medical problems, medications, allergies, habits, prior operations and hospitalizations, and family history. This meeting should also include a physical examination, since it is imperative that every surgeon personally examine every patient on whom he or she plans to operate. Certain findings, such as the presence and locations of previous abdominal scars or current hernias, or the identification of new findings such as a heart murmur, may mandate further evaluation or alter the surgical approach. It is always better to have this information beforehand than to be surprised at the time of surgery. The physical exam should include a height, weight, and calculation of a BMI. (If the surgeon does not calculate the BMI or know how to use it in determining your appropriateness for WLS, find another surgeon!!)

Nutritional Assessment: It is also a good idea for patients to be assessed by a dietitian. This need not be done at the initial visit but should be done at some time before surgery. The dietitian can obtain information about eating habits and patterns, including a measure of the number and source of calories consumed, which serves as a baseline. The dietitian can also screen for serious eating disorders, such as anorexia, and bulimia (bingeing, purging). These conditions may disqualify patients from surgery. If uncontrolled, eating disorders can cause physical harm after surgery by introducing huge amounts of food into the small stomach pouch. When eating disorders are identified, patients should be referred for appropriate treatment until the condition is under control, at which time surgery can again be considered.

Psychological Screening: The question of psychological screening is controversial. Patients often feel insulted or demeaned at the suggestion that they undergo an evaluation with a licensed clinical psychologist, social worker, or a psychiatrist. However, the goal of treatment is to provide the patient with the best outcome from surgery. If someone had a history of heart disease, it would be negligent for the surgeon not to ascertain the opinion of the treating cardiologist or obtain a consultation if there was no cardiologist. By the same token, if someone has a history of clinical depression or other psychological disorder and he or she is seeing a mental-health professional, then it would be negligent to proceed to surgery without obtaining his or her opinion or otherwise requesting a consultation. Many times, the consulting mental-health professional concludes that the patient has no psychological problem or that the problems are under control. Occasionally, however, a serious issue is identified that requires treatment. Many insurance carriers require a pre-operative psychological evaluation and will not authorize WLS without one. Most bariatric surgeons may not feel that routine psychological consultations are necessary, because the surgeon, along with a dietitian, can adequately screen patients for eating disorders. But when insurance carriers have particular requirements, there is little choice.

At the conclusion of the initial consultation, the surgeon, or his or her staff, should review the type of procedure proposed, explaining in layman's terms what he or she will do, how it works, and what results to expect. Sometimes, additional tests or consultations may be ordered to better evaluate the patient's condition and suitability for surgery.

Commonly Requested Tests

Blood tests: Blood chemistries, blood counts, a test of clotting ability, and a urinalysis are routinely performed before any major surgery. Other tests in obese patients that might be beneficial include: thyroid or adrenal-hormone tests (to rule out certain treatable hormone problems as the cause of the obesity), serum insulin or hemoglobin A_1C (which are extremely sensitive screening tests for diabetes), a complete lipid profile (to rule out blood-lipid abnormalities), and an arterial blood gas (ABG, a sample of blood drawn from an artery to measure the level of oxygen in the blood and help assess the risk from anesthesia).

Chest X Rays: Patients with severe obesity often have an enlarged heart and accompanying pulmonary problems. A screening chest X ray can provide valuable baseline information about the condition of the heart and lungs.

Upper-GI Series: Patients who have already had WLS should have an upper-gastrointestinal (upper-GI) series to help the surgeon visualize exactly what was done during the previous operation and better plan the current procedure. A routine upper-GI before all WLS is not necessary. In patients with a history of ulcer disease or severe reflux esophagitis, it might also provide useful information. However, these conditions are probably better evaluated by endoscopy (seen directly through a lighted scope passed into the stomach and intestine).

Electrocardiogram (ECG): Patients with severe obesity often have underlying cardiac problems that predispose them to sudden cardiac death. A screening ECG can detect an abnormality that requires further evaluation.

Sleep Study: Obstructive sleep apnea and the obesity hypoventilation syndrome are among the most dangerous complications of severe obesity. Patients with symptoms of these disorders, such as snoring, daytime sleepiness, and observed periods in which they stop breathing, should have a sleep study to rule out sleep apnea. This type of screening may be performed at home or through a formal sleep study, which requires an overnight stay in the hospital.

Screening for Gallstones: There is a strong relationship between obesity and gallstones and a high incidence of gallbladder attacks during weight loss in patients with gallstones. For this reason, it is customary for patients to be screened for gallstones before WLS. This evaluation is usually done with an ultrasound, which is not painful and does not expose the individual to radiation. Simply feeling the gallbladder at the time of surgery is extremely inaccurate and an unreliable technique for detecting gallstones. Patients who have documented gallstones should have their gallbladder removed (cholecystectomy) at the time of surgery.

Specialist Consultations: Consultations with specialists are desirable before surgery to more thoroughly evaluate certain conditions or get them under better control. Areas often evaluated include: cardiology, pulmonary medicine, endocrinology, psychiatry, and sleep medicine. In patients who need endoscopy for evaluation of ulcer disease or severe reflux esophagitis, consultation with a gastroenterologist (GI specialist) will be necessary if the surgeon does not perform this test.

For patients with serious associated medical problems, who might be at higher than usual risk for WLS, it is extremely useful for the patient to be evaluated by the anesthesiologist before surgery. The role of the anesthesiologist is critical in successfully performing WLS. Consultation with an anesthesiologist before-hand can often save valuable time on the day of surgery should any questions or problems arise. Talking with the anesthesiologist can also allay a patient's fears about being put to sleep by allowing the physician to explain the procedure step-by-step. Losing consciousness is scary for most patients, and knowing and trusting who is going to "put you under" can be extremely reassuring.

It is customary for most laboratory tests and X rays to be obtained prior to admission to the hospital, usually during the week before surgery. This allows for the results to be reviewed and any potential problems identified and corrected.

The Night Before Surgery

Aspiration of stomach contents into the lungs can cause pneumonia. For this reason, it is advisable for the stomach to be empty of food or liquids before surgery, which usually takes about six to eight hours after eating. Because most operations are scheduled early in the day, patients are usually told to avoid eating or drinking after midnight on the night before the operation. Occasionally, patients are advised to take certain medications, such as blood-pressure pills, early in the morning with only a sip of water.

In addition, it may be advisable to shower with an antiseptic soap, which can help decrease the bacterial count on the skin, especially in regions such as the umbilicus (belly button) or within skin creases that are otherwise difficult to clean. Cleansing in this manner can help reduce the chances of wound infections.

Some surgeons may prescribe a "bowel prep" for their patients, which is a regimen designed to clean the intestine of stool. Bowel preps typically involve drinking one gallon of a solution that does not get absorbed from the intestine into the body and hence passes through the entire intestinal tract, flushing the stool out of the colon. Bowel preps were actually developed for colon surgery, where their use is associated with a lower risk of wound infections, and to prepare the bowel for procedures such as colonoscopy, where stool would interfere with the examiner's ability to see the colon. Bowel preps are not needed for gastric or small-intestinal surgery, because the bacterial content of these areas is much lower than in the colon and the risk of infection is less.

WHAT TO EXPECT IN THE HOSPITAL (PERI-OPERATIVELY)

The care I got was exceptional. They had state-of-the-art equipment for people my size. I didn't have to be embarrassed by not fitting into a wheelchair. The nurses were very kind to me. All in all, considering it was a hospital, it was pretty nice.

Sharyn J., 44, 447 lbs. pre-op; 293 lbs. 2½ years post-op

I was so happy that I didn't have to stay in the intensive-care unit. The sounds of all the machines in that place make me nervous. My family was with me most of the time, which kept me fairly calm.

Michael S., 36, 384 lbs. pre-op; 237 lbs. 21 months post-op

Most patients undergoing WLS are admitted to the hospital on the morning of the operation. Occasionally, patients with serious underlying illnesses or those on blood thinners are admitted the day before surgery. Most hospitals have patients report to their admission-day or same-day-surgery centers one to two hours before the scheduled time of surgery.

Even though patients will typically be instructed to stop eating and drinking by midnight the night before surgery, they might still need to take certain medications early on the morning of surgery. In these cases, make sure you get specific instructions beforehand. It is a good idea to bring all medications to the hospital in case any questions arise at the last minute.

A number of procedures will be done once the patient arrives at the hospital so that the operation can proceed smoothly. Some of these treatments are standard and every surgeon does them, others are not, and surgeons differ in what they consider essential for each patient.

Intravenous (IV): All patients having any major surgery require an IV for the administration of fluids and drugs. This can usually be placed in an arm. Occasionally, placement is difficult in obese patients, and placement of special IVs in larger, central veins is necessary. These larger IVs, called CVPs, are typically inserted under the collarbone.

Arterial Line (A-Line): An arterial line is like an IV that is placed into an artery, usually in the wrist. It provides a constant measurement of blood pressure during the operation and allows the anesthesiologist to easily sample the blood in order to monitor the level of oxygen in it. There is some risk associated with the use of an arterial line. If a clot develops, the blood flow to the hand could be seriously impaired. For this reason, only a minority of surgeons and anesthesiologists use these routinely during WLS. Instead, most use them selectively in patients with more serious problems, such as heart disease or sleep apnea.

Urinary Catheter (Foley catheter): A urinary catheter is a plastic tube inserted into the bladder, used to drain the urine into a collection bag. This allows the doctors to measure the exact amount of urine made, which provides them with information about how well the heart and kidneys are functioning. Such information is valuable in complex cases, when it is difficult to assess cardiac function using ordinary clinical parameters, like blood pressure and heart rate. The risk in using a urinary catheter is that patients become more susceptible to urinary-tract infections, which prolong their hospitalization and slow their recovery. Although many bariatric surgeons routinely use urinary catheters during and after WLS, I have only rarely found them necessary and do not routinely use them in my practice. Also, patients who are not catheterized are able to get out of bed to use the bathroom after surgery, which provides needed exercise.

Antibiotics: All operations in which the stomach, small intestine, or colon are opened carry a risk of wound infection. In WLS, infection rates as high as 15 percent have been reported. The threat of infection can be dramatically reduced by giving antibiotics for the twenty-four-hour period surrounding surgery, being careful to begin before the operation (prophylactic antibiotics). All patients having WLS should receive prophylactic antibiotics.

Usually, a penicillin-like drug called cefazolin is used, and in cases where the patient is allergic to penicillin, an appropriate substitute is administered. In my last 1,000 cases, I changed my method of skin closure from staples to a subcuticular (plastic-surgery-type stitch) with a drain, which reduced my wound-infection rate from about 10 percent to 2 percent.

Preventive Measures for Blood Clots: The development of blood clots in the major veins of the legs and pelvis (deep vein thrombosis), which can then break into smaller clots that can travel to the lungs (pulmonary emboli), is a serious concern. Although all people undergoing major surgery are at risk for these, the risk is much higher in severely obese patients. Blood clots in the veins can cause pain, chronic swelling, skin changes, and ulcers, but it is the fear of pulmonary emboli, which can be fatal, that is the most serious concern. For this reason, most surgeons performing WLS employ preventive measures to reduce this threat.

These preventive methods consist of the use of drugs and/or mechanical devices. The drug most commonly used is called heparin. It is usually given by injection into the thigh or abdominal wall twice a day and should be started before surgery. The mechanical devices that patients sometimes call "booties" are pneumatic compression stockings and are similar to blood-pressure cuffs. They are placed on the legs and thighs and connected to a machine that inflates and intermittently deflates. These stockings prevent clots from forming by maintaining circulation in the veins. At the present, there is no strong scientific information to favor the use of either method by itself or the combination, and surgeons have their own preferences.

Nasogastric Tube (NG Tube): A nasogastric tube is a plastic-like tube that is passed through the nose, down the esophagus, and lodges in the stomach or small intestine. It is often used after upper-abdominal or stomach surgery to suck juices or air out of the stomach, thus preventing swelling of the stomach or intestine that could tear the sutures or staples. In the past, the use of NG tubes was routine after major abdominal surgery. However, in the past ten years, the use of these tubes has become optional as research has shown that patients tolerate many operations without needing them. In my practice, I no longer routinely leave a nasogastric tube in place after WLS. Surgeons who employ NG tubes after weight loss procedures usually remove them after an X ray that shows there is no leak.

Many patients fear the NG tube. However, if your surgeon requires the NG tube, be reassured that it is usually inserted after you are asleep. Although it might feel slightly uncomfortable, it doesn't hurt and probably won't bother you at all. Removal of the tube is somewhat unpleasant but usually quick. Most patients report that their fear of the NG tube was unfounded.

Checking for Leaks: A leak is a serious complication because it often requires another operation to repair it and prolongs the hospitalization and recovery. Also, if a leak is not detected and repaired quickly, it can cause severe infection, resulting in damage to the lungs, kidneys, and other organs, and occasionally death. For this reason, most surgeons routinely check for leaks during the operation. In addition, many also look for leaks postoperatively with an upper-GI X ray. This requires the patient to swallow gastrograffin, which might be unpleasant but is not painful. These tests are usually performed on the first or second morning after surgery. If the X ray shows no leak, the NG tube, if present, is removed and the patient is usually started on liquids.

Drains: Drains are tubes that are placed in a body cavity to drain fluid that accumulates to the outside. In WLS, many surgeons will place a drain near the stomach so that if a leak occurs, the fluid from the stomach will hopefully be sucked out of the body, avoiding the formation of a fluid collection or abscess, and possibly another operation.

Pain: All operations cause pain, whether performed open or laparoscopically. Numerous medications, usually narcotics like morphine or Demerol, are available to control it. Initially, these drugs are given by vein or injection because they are more effective when administered by these routes when patients are not yet eating or drinking. A popular method is called *patient-controlled analgesia*, or PCA, in which the drug, usually morphine or Demerol, is administered at a constant rate by a pump with the dosage controlled by the patient. Many surgeons routinely employ the PCA pump; if yours does not, you can certainly inquire about it. Once eating and drinking are permitted, the transition is made to oral medications, often containing codeine. As mentioned earlier, aspirin and aspirin-like drugs (NSAIDs) can cause stomach upset and ulcers and should be avoided. Acetaminophen (Tylenol) does not produce these side effects and is permitted.

Admission to the ICU: Patients undergoing WLS frequently have many potentially life-threatening medical problems. Occasionally, these can be severe enough to mandate admission to the intensive-care unit after surgery for closer monitoring of heart and lung function. However, routine admission to the ICU is probably not necessary, and most surgeons do not require it.

WHAT TO EXPECT AFTER YOU GO HOME (POST-OPERATIVELY)

I was really glad that I had arranged for my mother to stay with me for the week following surgery. I was pretty much able to take care of myself, but it was nice to be babied. I took naps in the afternoon for most of that week, and she watched the kids.

Heather M., 42, 388 lbs. pre-op; 225 lbs. 5 years post-op

My sister flew in from Ohio to care for me. I felt pretty good most of the time, so we did some really great catching up.

Renee B., 37, 278 lbs. pre-op; 202 lbs. 9 months post-op

I had a urinary-tract infection after my operation, which made me feel really lousy. After the antibiotics started to kick in, I began feeling a lot better.

Diana W., 45, 441 lbs. pre-op; 274 lbs. 2 years post-op

I went back to work only two weeks after my surgery on a part-time basis. It felt great to be out in the world again. I did tire easily for a while—but I guess that's the case after any major surgery.

James P., 44, 359 lbs. pre-op; 263 lbs. 18 months post-op

Recovery from all types of major surgery, including WLS, requires several weeks. During this period, improvement will occur in several areas, including physical well-being, activity level, and diet.

Physical Well-Being: The predominant symptom experienced during this phase is fatigue. Patients become easily tired with even mild activity. Improvement is gradual, and normal levels of stamina return by four to six weeks. Return of strength may be faster after laparoscopic surgery; however, there is much individual variation.

Activity Level and Returning to Work: Returning to work is dependent upon the speed of each person's recovery and the nature of their work. If people feel well and do not engage in physically demanding work, they may return as early as one or two weeks after surgery. In some cases, it may be wise to return on a part-time basis for a while. The more physically demanding the work, the longer the delay should be, with the most strenuous jobs requiring six to eight weeks for the incision to be fully healed to reduce the chance of developing a hernia in the incision. Although the incisions utilized in laparoscopy are smaller than with open surgery, there is still a risk of hernia.

Dietary Progression: Dietary progression after WLS varies, based on the type of procedure and the personal preference of the surgeon. Several approaches to dietary management exist, and most are equally valid.

The restrictive operations—RYGB, VBG, and gastric banding—act by reducing food intake. They each leave very small stomach pouches, which only tolerate frequent small meals. Most surgeons recommend liquids, blenderized, or soft foods for the first four weeks or so after surgery. Emphasis should be on consuming foods high in protein, such as dairy products, and maintaining good hydration by drinking between two and three quarts of liquid a day.

The malabsorptive procedures, such as BPD or DS, cause

weight loss by limiting absorption of nutrients, not by reducing intake. Patients who undergo these procedures have greater stomach capacities and are rapidly progressed to pureed and soft foods for three weeks, after which they can eat whatever they want.

Medications: Most patients leave the hospital after WLS with prescriptions for a variety of medications. Pain medication, usually a codeine derivative, is routine. Often, these stronger pills can be alternated with acetaminophen if pain is not severe. Vitamins are also frequently recommended after all types of WLS, although they are needed more after the malabsorptive procedures and RYGB. Individuals with intact gallbladders should be given Actigall or Urso250 in order to prevent the formation of gallstones with weight loss. Some surgeons also prescribe H_2-blockers or proton pump inhibitors to try to prevent marginal-ulcer formation.

12

HANDLING PRE-OP JITTERS

BEING NERVOUS IS NORMAL

Being nervous before surgery is perfectly normal. In fact, I worry more about people who are not concerned. After all, surgery is associated with risks and, despite the fact that the operation may be in the best interest of the patient's health, complications can occur.

Tara, age 22 and 350 pounds, expresses the pre-op jitters perfectly:

I was really nervous the night before my surgery. Unable to fall asleep, my heart raced and my mind reeled with thoughts about the following morning. Fleetingly, I worried about dying and how my death would affect those I love. Mostly, I agonized about whether or not I was making the right decision. Would the results of the operation be worth all of the pain I would have to go through? I can't tell anyone who is considering WLS not to worry. There are risks involved. I was really terrified. I understand now that my anxiety was normal. I'm grateful my fears didn't get the best of me and cause me to back out. Despite all of my anxieties, I persevered—and I'm glad that I did.

GET SUPPORT

I was really nervous telling my family about this operation. They live clear across the country, and I could have informed them after the fact. However, I'm happy that I bit the bullet and told the truth.

They surprised me by being very supportive. My mother and sister flew in to be with me. I should have given them more credit.

Leslie L., 32, 319 lbs. pre-op; 158 lbs. 3½ years post-op

I got a great deal of support from my friends on-line—especially the veterans. They really gave me an idea of what I would be going through. There is no substitute for talking to people who are in the same boat.

Raymond V., 43, 332 lbs. pre-op; 196 lbs. 22 months post-op

Once you are committed to having surgery, there are a number of steps you can take to get over the pre-op jitters:

Join an On-Line Support Group: If you have a computer, go onto the Internet and join OSSG@egroups.com or visit Carnie Wilson's support group at www.spotlighthealth.com and click on *morbid obesity.* If you don't own a computer, you can join these groups by using the computer at your local library and signing up for a free e-mail account at Hotmail.com or Yahoo.com. Reading the stories about people like yourself who have had surgery (and only wished they'd done it sooner) is enormously reassuring.

Visit Your Doctor's Support Group: While you wait, visit your doctor's support group or any other group in your area. There is no substitute for meeting people who have gone through this surgery, talking to them about their experiences, and getting your questions answered firsthand. If there is no support group near you, ask your doctor for the telephone numbers of some post-op patients and call them. Try to see if you "click" with one of them, and ask if they would mind a phone call when you're feeling low. Most post-op patients are eager to share their success with others and will be happy to offer telephone encouragement when you need it.

Do Research and More Research: The more information you have, the better you will feel. The fact is that gastric bypass is as safe as other major gastrointestinal operations. If you have questions about any aspect of the procedure, do not hesitate to ask your doctor. You need to have total confidence in your surgeon. There is an enormous amount of information about bariatric surgery available on the Web. (See website list in Appendix A.) Again, the librarian at your local library will show you how to access these sites if you don't have a computer.

Use Self-Help Books and Relaxation Tapes. Many of these are available at bookstores or on the Internet at on-line bookstores like Amazon.com, Barnes&Noble.com, or Powells.com (see Appendix A).

Talk to Your Anesthesiologist. Many people are terrified of being unconscious and never waking up, or have had negative experiences in the past with anesthesia. Discussing these concerns with the anesthesiologist ahead of time can allay many of these fears.

Analyze Your Fears One at a Time. Avoid "awfulizing" by lumping all of your fears into one big basket. Research the reality of that particular fear, because the chances are you've exaggerated it. For example, many pre-op patients are afraid of failing at this weight loss method, just like they've failed at everything they've tried in the past. However, research shows that the vast majority of patients who have WLS are successful at losing weight and maintaining it.

Here are some other common fears:

Fear of the Unknown: This is a natural emotion. The anxieties that many pre-op patients express are real and need validation but should not be allowed to become a barrier to success.

Fear of Failure: Many previous weight loss attempts have been unsuccessful, and the ugly thought that this will be another failed attempt may creep into your mind. Research shows that 75 percent of patients lose an average of 65 percent of their excess weight and keep most of it off. A positive frame of mind, lifestyle changes, and surgery are the best tools to ensure success. Visualize yourself with 65 percent of your excess weight lost, and think about how you will look and feel. Make a list of all the reasons why surgery is different from any other attempt you have made in the past and another list of the personal goals you want to accomplish by undergoing surgery. Add to the list anytime you can. Keep it at hand and look at it each time you need to refresh your psyche.

Fear of Pain and a Lengthy Recovery: Speak to your surgeon about pain management and the expected length of recovery. Prepare yourself mentally for some physical discomfort, which is a normal part of the healing process. Think about how you have handled pain in the past, what was successful in reducing it and what was not. Turn your fear into hope. Try to remember that this will be a temporary situation; each day that passes post-operatively will bring you closer to the life you want and include less pain. Close your eyes for a moment; think about your life now and the pain you endure on a daily basis. Visualize what life will be like without pain. That is the goal you want to achieve.

Fear of Dumping, Vomiting, or Not Being Able to Eat: Speak with your surgeon and the dietitian in advance of surgery and ask their advice on how to adjust the "new eating regime" so you will not only lose unwanted weight but also keep your body nourished and healthy. Prepare your house with foods you will eat after surgery, and clean the refrigerator and cabinets of "danger and trigger" foods that you will no longer eat. Early in your recovery process keep a food diary, which includes information about how much you ate and how you felt after eating. This information, together with the dietitian, will help you to develop a successful food plan. It may seem like a challenge initially, but with patience you will adjust to your new way of eating, and it will be a comforting, daily reminder that your body will no longer tolerate the large amounts of food that led you to the pains of obesity.

Fear of Hunger: Hunger, both physical and psychological, comes in many forms. The surgical procedure will address the physical hunger for the most part, but more introspective work needs to be done to cope with the psychological hunger and what that means to you. Seeking a therapist experienced in treatment of WLS patients can be helpful both before and after surgery. Your therapist can not only help with fears and anxieties pre-op, but also work with you after surgery as you adjust your thoughts about hunger and realize that hunger is not an enemy to be feared. You will need to develop new strategies to call upon when your old coping pattern included overeating.

Although you will not feel hunger in the early weeks and even months post-op, you may begin to experience it as you normalize your life. Some initial helpful tips are: Accept that you will feel hunger at times and know, in advance, how you will handle it. Try to eat low-calorie foods, exercise, go for a drive, meditate, or call a friend, and eventually the sensation will pass. It's okay to feel hunger. Normal-weight people experience it regularly. Try acknowledging your hunger and making a conscious decision as to when and what to eat. Remaining in control of the hunger is paramount.

Don't panic. You may have days that you are more hungry than others, and that is normal. Panic will only interfere with your ability to see your weight loss as a long-term process that involves changing behaviors.

Fear of Death: All surgery comes with risks, but so does obesity. Undergoing this operation means taking a short-term risk, but the long-term benefits outweigh the risk for most patients. Regardless of the benefits, facing the possibility of death is scary, and no words can disguise the fear and anguish. There is no magical visualization that eliminates the fear of dying. You need to tap into your innermost resources to help alleviate the anxiety associated with the fear. Do whatever it is that helps you overcome difficulties in your life: Seek spiritual or psychological support; speak with family and friends; explore the Internet for information and peers; see a therapist or counselor. But, most important, allow yourself to be afraid and not let the fear paralyze your thoughts and actions.

I must be the luckiest person on the face of the planet. My therapist had WLS surgery, so she understood exactly what I was going through. I'm not sure how I would have made it without her.

Val G., 28, 374 lbs. pre-op; 227 lbs. 4 years post-op

I had seen a therapist after the death of my husband. She really helped me with the grieving process. It was only natural for me to turn to her when I needed help making the decision about whether or not to have WLS. Talking it through with my therapist—listing and discussing all of the pros and cons of surgery—really helped me figure out what to do. It was such a relief to talk to someone so nonjudgmental about what I planned to do. I really felt understood and supported and that I made an informed decision.

Stephanie R., 46, 356 lbs. pre-op; 233 lbs. 2 years post-op

Write down all the reasons you want to lose 100 pounds or more and read your answers when you're feeling nervous. (This list originally appeared on OSSG.)

101 reasons to lose 100 lbs.

1. To feel good about yourself
2. To have GREAT sex! :)
3. So you won't think people are laughing or talking about you
4. To buy clothes in a normal store that are actually stylish and fit correctly
5. To have more energy
6. To be able to tie your shoes and paint your toenails
7. To be able to sit on a floor and get up gracefully
8. To wear a bathing suit
9. To cross your legs
10. To fit into an airline, theater, bus, or whatever seat without spilling over and without having to see "that look" from the person who has to sit beside you
11. So your ankles won't swell
12. To fit into a booth at any restaurant
13. To not need an extension to a seat belt on an airplane and to have the tray table not balance on your belly
14. To not worry about being hit by the air bag in your car during an accident because you have to sit so close to it
15. To not turn beet red after moderate exertion
16. To be able to pick something up off the floor
17. To buy panty hose that fit
18. To go to an amusement park and ride the rides
19. To be able to sit in any chair without worrying about breaking it

20. To not have to apologize when caught in a narrow aisle and have someone need to get by
21. To go dancing, skydiving, bungee jumping
22. To be able to go horseback riding or ride a bike
23. To not worry about rashes and sweating in unreachable places
24. To not have to listen to "caring" people ask why you don't diet or, worse still, say, "Gee, you have such a pretty face"
25. To not worry about spilling food, sauces, or gravy down the front of your blouse, dress, or shirt when you're eating
26. To not have to think up some excuse for not doing something because you know your weight will impede you
27. To not have your belly hit the steering wheel and to be able to fit comfortably in the driver's seat
28. To have a bra fit comfortably and to be able to buy underwear at Victoria's Secret rather than at "Tubby the Underwear Guy"
29. To not have to worry about the weight limit of step stools, ladders, motorcycles, exercise equipment, etc.
30. To not get stuck in a turnstile
31. To not wake up feeling achy in your back or to have ache-free legs and feet
32. So the bathroom scale won't creak and groan when you step on it
33. To be able to leave the tablecloth on the table at a restaurant instead of dragging it with you when you get up
34. So you won't look the other way when you see yourself in a monitor where they have security cameras
35. To never be embarrassed about your size
36. To not count walking to the refrigerator as daily exercise
37. To not have to wait for the handicapped bathroom stalls when there are plenty of other stalls available
38. To not be more out of shape than senior citizens
39. To not break the toilet seat when leaning to one side
40. To be able to put on wedding rings again
41. To try to make a double chin and fail
42. To buy clothing bargains that fit for the next year

43. To not have to worry about plastic zippers or having your pants burst open
44. To wear normal waistbands rather than elastic
45. To wear knee socks correctly instead of worn like slouches
46. To look good in a T-shirt
47. To try on slacks or jeans and have the pant leg actually fit over your leg
48. To be able to get close to the sink and not come away with a wet belly
49. To get out of a stuffed chair gracefully and not look down to see if the chair has come up with you
50. To not worry if the hairdresser's smock will fit
51. To not be self-conscious about eating in front of others
52. To not be afraid to ask which hairstyle suits your face
53. To not have people checking you out after looking in your grocery cart
54. To buy an item of clothing without an X in it
55. To have your friends not be embarrassed to be seen with you
56. To get promoted, hired, or close that sale
57. To wear pants that stay up because your waist is smaller than your butt
58. No more boobs! (This is for the guys!)
59. To wear shorts or tank tops without fear of arrest or grossing out others
60. To see your cholesterol plunge
61. To successfully flirt
62. To not worry about how to get in and out of the backseat in a two-door car
63. To wear "One size fits all" that fits you too
64. To have a lap
65. To not have the car you are riding in slant in your direction
66. To be able to use toilet paper as it was meant to be used and not to have to invent ways to "get the job done.":)
67. To not have to watch TV news reports on fat people in hopes that you haven't been caught on camera

68. To be able to get between cars in a parking lot without wiping the dust off with your belly and your butt
69. To not experience chafing of the upper thighs
70. So that the cloth in the thigh area doesn't wear away long before the rest of the slacks do
71. To meet a friend on-line and not be horrified to have to send a picture of yourself
72. To not take fat references and fat jokes personally
73. To know you can go anywhere because wherever you sit you can be comfortable and look at ease
74. To shop at the mall and not have your back ache from lugging your huge butt and stomach around
75. To be able to stand still carrying nothing and still look poised
76. To be able to cross your arms on your chest without them resting on your stomach!
77. To have your feet get smaller
78. To use your mouth to taste and chew food rather than as just a route to get the food from your lips to your stomach
79. To see your blood pressure return to normal
80. To see your blood sugar return to normal
81. To be able to borrow a coworker's jacket for an important impromptu meeting
82. To meet someone for the first time and their eyes don't pop out of their head with amazement . . . because they never knew you were so fat
83. To see your reflection in a mirror or store window without turning away
84. To wear a watch with a regular-length band
85. To not pee when you cough or sneeze
86. To not mind getting your picture taken
87. To not avoid going to the doctor because you have to get "weighed in"
88. To wake up each morning feeling energized and ready to go
89. To not even worry about squeezing into small spaces
90. To not have to enter an elevator and check the weight limit

91. To look in your closet and have problems deciding which stylish outfit to wear to work since you have so many that look good and fit well
92. To not have to lie perfectly still in bed at night for fear of breaking the bed
93. To buy tie shoes instead of slip-ons
94. To be able to walk any distance without resting on a bench
95. To look forward to shopping and just trying on clothes
96. To be able to drive by any fast-food place without salivating
97. To be able to shop at the same store for food instead of having to remember where you shopped last night for the junk food so you can avoid that store for a few days
98. To not feel lower than low when an innocent child remarks about your size
99. To not constantly be thinking of where your next morsel of food is coming from
100. To not get heartburn when you lie down
101. And the best reason to lose 100 pounds . . .

BECAUSE YOU'RE WORTH IT!

13

EATING AGAIN AFTER WEIGHT LOSS SURGERY

As you begin eating again, it is important to remember that changes are necessary in how you eat, how much you eat, and what you eat after WLS.

GENERAL GUIDELINES FOR EATING AFTER WEIGHT LOSS SURGERY

Gastric Bypass Surgery and Gastroplasty

Many patients are concerned or confused about eating after having a gastric bypass or gastroplasty. Here are some guidelines that will help.

You will be able to eat regular food again; however, it may take several weeks. During that time your diet will progress from soft foods, such as yogurt, cottage cheese, soup, and applesauce, to more-solid foods such as vegetables, pasta, fish, and meat. (It may take longer to tolerate solid foods after gastroplasty than gastric bypass.)

The progression to solid foods is sometimes tricky and involves a lot of trial and error. Do not be discouraged. If you find that you do not tolerate a particular food, wait a week and try it again. You *will* be able to eat most of the foods you ate before the surgery.

It is common to experience occasional vomiting, especially early on. Vomiting is often caused by trying to eat too much at one time or eating too quickly. As you learn to adjust your eating habits, it should become less of a problem.

You may not feel hungry or want to eat. Many people report that they no longer crave food and in fact have to be prodded and reminded to eat. It is important to eat in order to recover from your surgery and stay healthy.

After a few months you will be back on a modified regular diet and even be able to eat in restaurants. There will be certain foods you need to avoid, and you will need to eat smaller portions.

As you begin eating, keep in mind:

The anatomy of your stomach and intestine is very different after gastric bypass and gastroplasty and requires that you make changes in the way you eat, how much you eat, and what you eat. Your native stomach before surgery was approximately the size of a football. Your new stomach (gastric pouch) is much smaller, approximately the size of a medium egg, and holds about one ounce. Also, the opening from your stomach pouch to the rest of the stomach (after gastroplasty) or small intestine (after gastric bypass) is about a half inch wide, the size of an index finger.

Eat and drink only *small quantities* at a time. Trying to eat or drink too much at one sitting can cause vomiting.

Chew your food well so that it can be digested more easily and pass freely out of the pouch into the intestine.

Eat and drink *slowly*. If the pouch gets full quickly, you may experience nausea, vomiting, and pain.

Focus on eating healthier foods. This is especially important because you will be eating less, so what you eat matters more.

Do not advance your diet too quickly. It takes about a month for your digestive system to adjust to the changes from the surgery. Be patient—you will be able to eat regular food again!

Dumping Syndrome After Gastric Bypass

Dumping syndrome is caused by certain foods leaving the stomach and entering the small intestine too quickly. It can occur after any operation that changes the way food is routed during digestion. The normal stomach has a valve called the pylorus, which regulates the amount and speed with which food passes into the small intestine. Gastric bypass reroutes food around the pylorus, so food passes directly through the gastric pouch to the small intestine without any hindrance.

Certain foods, such as sugars, high-fat foods, and simple carbohydrates, absorb water and tend to produce symptoms that may include light-headedness, cold sweats, abdominal cramps, and diarrhea. The light-headedness and sweats are related to low blood sugar, similar to those that occur during an insulin reaction.

In addition to not eating sugars and dense fats, dumping can be avoided by eating six small meals per day, choosing foods high in protein content, drinking between meals instead of during meals, eating slowly, and resting a bit before getting up after eating. Our research has shown that most people find that sweets taste sweeter after gastric bypass surgery, so much so that many prefer to avoid sweets altogether. This decreases their chances of experiencing the dumping syndrome. Dumping syndrome does not occur after gastroplasty.

DIETARY PROGRESSION AFTER GASTRIC BYPASS AND GASTROPLASTY

Step I: Soft Diet (follow for about 2 weeks after surgery)
- During the initial 2 weeks after surgery, your diet will consist of mainly soft foods. Because your stomach pouch is small, the portions will be very small, making it necessary to eat at least six times per day.
- It is important to drink at least 2 quarts (8 cups) of liquids per day in order to prevent dehydration and constipation. This can be water, diluted fruit juice, sugar-free iced tea, sugar-free soft drinks, or milk.
- After 2 weeks, you will be able to begin adding solid foods to your diet.

Guidelines for Soft Diet
Warning: This diet does not contain enough calories, protein, vitamins, and minerals. Use only on the advice of your doctor for up to 4 weeks after gastric bypass surgery. It is not recommended for general weight loss.

- Your meals will consist of liquids and soft foods.

- The liquids will include water, diluted fruit juice, sugar-free drinks (unsweetened tea, unsweetened coffee, diet soda, sugar-free Kool-Aid, Crystal Light, etc.). In order to maximize protein intake, it may be best to drink between meals. Sugar-free Popsicles and sugar-free gelatin may also be used between meals.

- Avoid carbonated beverages. Some people will have discomfort and bloating from them.

- The soft foods may include cottage cheese, yogurt, eggs, soup, applesauce, and pureed vegetables.

- Take 2 chewable children's or adult vitamins (such as Flintstones Complete) every day. This will help prevent vitamin and mineral deficiencies.

- Take vitamins with your liquid meals. Do not drink coffee, tea, or diet cola with meals. These drinks may decrease the amount of vitamins your body absorbs.

- Eat at least 6 times a day. The amount you will be able to eat at one time is very small. You will need to eat many small meals to try to meet your Recommended Daily Allowances (RDA) for protein, vitamins, and minerals.

- Choose one item from the meat or milk group at each meal. These foods are high in protein. Protein helps your body heal after surgery.

- Avoid beverages that contain alcohol.

- Choose sugar-free chewing gum rather than sweetened. *Do not swallow it*.

- Blend all foods until smooth. The food should not have lumps, seeds, or small pieces.

- Drink at least 2 quarts of water or low-calorie liquid per day between meals.

- Sip liquid meals slowly. Drink 6 ounces, or ¾ cup, over 20 to 30 minutes.

- Record the foods you eat and the amounts for at least 2 to 3 days. Bring this with you to your next appointment with the dietitian. The dietitian will calculate the amount of calories and protein you are eating.

How to Blend Foods

- Cut foods into small pieces.

- Place food in blender or food processor.

- Add liquid such as broth, juice, or milk.

- Blend or puree until smooth.

- Strain foods that do not blend to a completely smooth consistency.

- Season foods to taste. You may want to avoid spicy seasonings (hot sauce, black pepper, cayenne pepper, red pepper, etc.).

Planning Meals

Use foods from the following groups to plan your meals:

Note: These are not the standard serving sizes recommended by the Food Guide Pyramid. They are specific for gastric bypass and gastroplasty patients.

Milk Group

Choose 3 to 4 servings from this food group each day because these items are good sources of protein and calcium:

½ c. skim or 1 percent low-fat milk
½ c. low-fat Lactaid milk
2 tbsp. nonfat dry milk powder
½ c. sugar-free, low-fat or nonfat yogurt (remove any pieces of fruit in yogurt)
½ pkg. sugar-free instant-breakfast drink
½ c. sugar-free pudding

Vegetable Group

Choose 2 servings from this food group each day because these items are good sources of vitamins, minerals, and fiber, and are low in calories:

½ c. vegetable juice (tomato, carrot, V8)

½ to 1 c. soft-cooked vegetables such as:

Asparagus	Eggplant	Beets
Green beans	Broccoli	Brussels sprouts
Spinach	Cauliflower	Cabbage
Tomato sauce	Carrots	Zucchini

Note: Cabbage, cauliflower, broccoli, and Brussels sprouts may cause abdominal discomfort and bloating. People having gastroplasty should avoid eating vegetable skins.

Fruit Group

Choose 2 servings from this food group each day because these items are good sources of vitamins, minerals, and fiber:

½ c. diluted, unsweetened fruit juice

½ to 1 c. blended, unsweetened fruit

Note: Full-strength (undiluted) fruit juice has more sugar, which may cause dumping syndrome. It is important to dilute juice by mixing ¼ cup juice and ¼ cup water. Avoid strained fruit desserts and junior or toddler foods that have added sugar.

Starch Group

Choose 2 servings from this food group each day because these items are good sources of energy, B vitamins, and iron (if fortified):

1 c. soup, any kind

½ c. cooked cereal such as:

Cream of Wheat, Cream of Rice

Oatmeal, grits

1 c. soft, starchy vegetable such as:

Creamed corn

Winter squash

Potatoes, any kind

Peas

Meat Group

Choose 4 servings from this food group each day because these items are good sources of protein, energy, B vitamins, and iron:

¼ c. egg substitute, cooked and blended

¼ c. low-fat cottage cheese

1 tbsp. smooth peanut butter

¼ c. water-packed tuna fish

1 oz. soft meat (beef, fish, turkey, chicken, veal, etc.)

Note: Many patients tolerate fish before they can tolerate chicken or beef. Progression after gastric bypass may be faster than after gastroplasty.

Fat Group

Choose 2 servings from this food group each day (you need some fat in your diet to maintain health):

1 tsp. regular margarine, butter, or oil

2 tsp. diet margarine

1 tbsp. low-fat mayonnaise or salad dressing

Sample Menu

Breakfast

½ c. skim milk	1 milk
½ c. Cream of Wheat	1 starch
2 tsp. diet margarine	1 fat

Mid-Morning

½ c. skim milk mixed with ½ pkg.	
sugar-free instant-breakfast drink	1 milk
¼ c. egg substitute	1 meat

Lunch

| ½–1 c. pureed vegetable with | 1 vegetable |
| ½ jar strained chicken | 1 meat |

Mid-Afternoon

½ c. low-fat cottage cheese	1 meat
½–1 c. fruit	1 fruit

Dinner

1 oz. soft-cooked beef with broth	1 meat
⅓ c. soft-cooked green beans	1 vegetable
⅓ c. mashed potatoes	1 starch
2 tsp. diet margarine	1 fat

Late Evening

½ c. sugar-free pudding or sugar-free, nonfat yogurt or skim milk	1 milk

In between meals you may eat sugar-free Popsicles, sugar-free gelatin, and drink sugar-free drinks.

Step II: Beginning Solid Foods
(start at 2 to 4 weeks after surgery)

- Begin by adding *one* new solid food daily.
- Be patient! Your tolerance will improve gradually.

General Guidelines

- Continue to eat 6 small liquid and soft-cooked meals each day, but add one solid food item per day. Initially, all new foods should be soft-cooked or canned. (Avoid any raw fruit or vegetable, nuts, popcorn, etc.)
- Record all new foods and any problems you have in your food diary. Bring this list to your next visit with the doctor and dietitian. If you have trouble with a new food, wait about a week before trying it again.
- Continue to take 2 chewable children's multivitamins each day. This will prevent vitamin and mineral deficiencies. You will advance to prenatal vitamins at about 6 weeks after surgery.

- Chew well so food is almost liquid before you swallow.
- Continue to eat small amounts, slowly. Eat about 2 tablespoons over 10 to 15 minutes.
- Continue to drink 2 quarts of water or other low-calorie fluid between meals.
- Avoid alcoholic beverages.
- It is better to have one place to eat (such as the kitchen table) and avoid reading or watching TV while eating. This helps you to enjoy your food, to concentrate on eating more slowly, and to realize when your stomach is full.

Steps for Adding Solid Foods

1. Try one small bite of the new food and chew well. Wait a few minutes. If there are no problems, repeat this process for the next 2 bites of food.
2. If after 3 bites there are no problems, finish eating the food.
3. If at any time you feel full, nauseated, or like vomiting, stop eating and rest. Take only clear liquids at the next meal and add soft food at the meal following the clear liquids. Try one solid food again the next day.

Planning Meals

Use foods from the following groups to plan your meals:

Milk Group

Choose 4 servings from this food group each day because these items are good sources of protein and calcium:

½–1 c. skim or 1 percent low-fat milk

½–1 c. low-fat, lactose-reduced milk

2 tbsp. nonfat dry milk powder

½ c. sugar-free, low-fat or nonfat yogurt

½ pkg. sugar-free instant-breakfast drink

½ c. sugar-free pudding

Vegetable Group

Choose 3 to 4 servings from this food group each day because these items are good sources of vitamins, minerals, and fiber, and are low in calories:

½ c. vegetable juice (tomato, carrot, V8)
½–1 c. soft-cooked vegetables such as:

Asparagus	Eggplant	Beets
Green beans	Broccoli	Greens
Brussels sprouts	Spinach	Cabbage
Tomato sauce	Carrots	Zucchini
Cauliflower		

Note: Cabbage, cauliflower, broccoli, and Brussels sprouts may cause abdominal discomfort and bloating. Avoid raw vegetables until 6 to 8 weeks after surgery.

Fruit Group

Choose 3 to 4 servings from this food group each day because these items are good sources of vitamins, minerals, and fiber:

½ c. diluted, unsweetened fruit juice
1 c. unsweetened canned or cooked fruit. Avoid raw fruits until 6 to 8 weeks after surgery.

Note: Full strength (undiluted) fruit juice has more sugar, which may cause dumping syndrome. It is important to dilute juice by mixing together ¼ c. juice and ¼ c. water. Avoid strained fruit desserts and junior or toddler foods. These foods have added sugar.

Starch Group

Choose 3 to 4 servings from this food group each day because these items are good sources of energy, B vitamins, and iron (if fortified):

1 c. soup, any kind
6 saltine crackers
½ c. cooked pasta or macaroni
1 c. cooked cereal such as:
Cream of Wheat, Cream of Rice, oatmeal, grits
¾ c. sweetened dry cereal such as:

Cheerios, Corn Flakes, Puffed Rice,
Puffed Wheat, Rice Krispies
1 c. cooked starchy vegetable such as:
Winter squash, potatoes, peas

Note: Avoid bread, rolls, and buns until 6 to 8 weeks after surgery. They are usually not tolerated well when eaten before that time. When ready to add bread, try toast first. Chew it well. At first you may only be able to eat ¼ to ½ slice of bread.

Meat Group

Choose 4 from this food group each day because these items are good sources of protein, energy, B vitamins, and iron:

1 egg
¼ c. egg substitute, cooked and blended
1 tbsp. smooth peanut butter
1 oz. low-fat luncheon meat
1 oz. low-fat mild cheese
¼ c. low-fat cottage cheese
1 oz. soft-cooked meat (fish, chicken in small pieces, beef, pork, turkey, veal, meat loaf)

Note: Meat must be very moist. Try tuna, ham, or chicken salad made with fat-free mayonnaise. Meat tenderizer may help with beef or pork. Fat-free gravy also may help. Chili is usually well tolerated.

Fat Group

Choose 2 to 3 servings from this food group each day:

1 tsp. butter, regular margarine, or oil
2 tsp. diet margarine
1 tbsp. low-fat mayonnaise or salad dressing

Sample Menu

Breakfast

1 scrambled egg	1 meat
1–2 tsp. diet margarine	1 fat
½ c. diluted orange juice	1 fruit

Mid-Morning

1 pkg. sugar-free instant-breakfast drink	2 milk
1 tbsp. smooth peanut butter	1 meat

Lunch

½ c. plain cooked noodles	1 starch
1 oz. chicken in small pieces	1 meat
2 tsp. diet margarine	1 fat

Mid-Afternoon

¼–½ c. low-fat cottage cheese	1 meat
1 c. diced peaches in their own juice	1 fruit

Dinner

1 c. soft-cooked green beans	1 vegetable
1 oz. tender cooked fish in small pieces	1 meat
½ c. soft-cooked potatoes	1 starch
2 tsp. diet margarine	1 fat

Late Evening

½ c. skim or 1 percent low-fat milk	1 milk
¾ c. Cheerios	1 starch

High-Protein Foods

Remember as you begin advancing the diet, try adding diced meats, poultry, and fish or low-fat cheese. Begin with small amounts and increase quantity as tolerated. (¼ c. = 2 oz.)

		Protein (g)	Calories
1 oz.	Tender cooked fish, chicken, beef, pork, or ground, diced, shredded meat	7	75
1	Low-fat hot dog	5	100
1 oz.	(1 slice) Low-fat lunch meat	7	75
1 oz.	(1 slice) Low-fat mild cheese, string cheese	7	80
½ c.	Low-fat cottage cheese	13	80
1	Cooked egg	7	100
½ c.	Beans (pinto, black, etc.)	7	110
½ c.	Chili	9	150

DIETARY PROGRESSION AFTER BILIO-PANCREATIC DIVERSION AND DUODENAL SWITCH

Patients should have fewer problems with eating after BPD or DS than after a gastric bypass or gastroplasty, because the stomach is larger. Also, with the DS modification the pyloric valve is retained, so dumping is avoided. Patients can be discharged from the hospital on soft food and rapidly advance to solids as tolerated. However, there are several important facts to keep in mind:

- You are at a higher risk for nutritional deficiencies than gastric bypass patients, because much more of the intestine has been bypassed and weight loss after BPD or DS is primarily caused by malabsorption. People who require regular medications, such as thyroid medication, may not be good candidates for BPD or DS, because medicine as well as food is malabsorbed.
- Avoid high-fat foods. The more fat you eat, the more diarrhea you'll have.
- Eat as much protein as you possibly can. If you can eat 80 to 120 grams of protein a day, you probably will not need supplements. However, if you cannot get this much protein in food, take protein supplements.
- Avoid sugars. People absorb 100 percent of sugars after both BPD or DS, but people who have had the DS modification are NOT at risk for the dumping syndrome. Drinking nondietetic sodas and eating cookies, cake, ice cream, and candy can lead to insufficient weight loss after DS.
- Take fat-soluble vitamins. *Good brand:* ADEKS by Scandipharm.
- Take calcium supplements: 1,500 to 2,000 mg of calcium per day.

TIPS ON PROTEIN AND VITAMIN SUPPLEMENTS FOR WLS PATIENTS

High-Protein Foods After WLS

- Protein is necessary for everyone, but it is especially important for those who have had gastric bypass surgery or BPD/DS. Adequate protein intake ensures proper healing of your incision and your new stomach pouch. It also promotes the maintenance of muscle mass during weight loss. Not enough protein in your diet results in poor healing, hair loss, and an overall decrease in energy.

- Because you will be eating smaller amounts with your new stomach pouch, it is important to choose foods that are high in protein, such as meat and dairy products. Try to include at least one serving from one of these groups at each meal and snack. Your protein needs are determined by your *desirable* body weight and should be about 1 gram per kg per day, or ½ gram per pound per day.

Food labels will provide the protein content of most foods. Here are some foods that are especially high in protein.

High-Protein Liquid and Blended Foods	Protein (g)	Calories
1 c. skim milk	8	90
1 c. sugar-free low-fat yogurt	8	90
½ c. nonfat cottage cheese	13	70
1 envelope sugar-free instant-breakfast with 1 c. skim milk	15	160
1 c. strained or blended cream soup made with skim milk	8	200
1 c. sugar-free pudding made with skim milk	10	110
½ c. egg substitute	10	50
2 tbsp. creamy peanut butter	9	190

Note: You can also increase the protein content of soft foods by adding powdered skim milk. One tablespoon adds 2 grams of protein yet only 28 calories. You can double the protein in milk by adding 1 cup of nonfat dry milk to 1 quart of skim milk (14 grams protein and 149 calories per 8 ounces).

High-Protein Liquids

Peanut Butter Shake—350 cal. & 20 g protein
(Makes about 1 c.)

¼ c. powdered skim milk
½ c. water
3 crushed ice cubes
1 tsp. imitation vanilla
1 pkg. artificial sweetener
2 tbsp. creamy peanut butter
¼ banana

Blend nonfat milk with water. Add peanut butter, blend until smooth. Add remaining ingredients. Blend until smooth.

Meal in a Glass—220 cal. & 15 g protein
(Makes about 1¼ c.)

1 c. skim milk
1 envelope sugar-free instant breakfast
¼ c. fresh raspberries, strawberries, or blueberries

Blend until smooth.

Vitamins Are Important—How and When to Take Them
- *Vitamins:* For the first six weeks, use chewable vitamins. Any standard children's chewable vitamin will do. Take two children's multivitamins a day (at different times—preferably with food).
- *Calcium:* Initially, take three chewable calcium carbonate tablets (such as Tums) per day with food. If you can tolerate the size of the pills, switch to calcium citrate eventually, because it is absorbed better. When able, increase to 1,500 to 2,000 mg calcium per day.
- *Iron:* Iron is absorbed best if taken on an empty stomach

with vitamin C. If you suffer from anemia pre- or post-op, take at least 150 mg a day of elemental iron.

Recommended: Niferex or Niferex Forte with B_{12} and folate. It's more easily absorbed and doesn't cause gastrointestinal problems. (If your insurance doesn't cover Niferex, order the generic, Fe-Tinic, from your pharmacist. It's less expensive.)

- *Vitamin B_{12}:* Take sublingual B_{12} (the type that dissolves under your tongue) to avoid deficiency.
- Vitamin B_{12} deficiencies may not show up until 9 months or one year after surgery, since it's stored in the body and takes time to be depleted. After 6 months, use 500 mcg of sublingual B_{12} per day.

SECRETS OF LONG-TERM SUCCESS: HOW WEIGHT LOSS SURGERY CAN CHANGE YOUR LIFE

Erica Manfred writes:

I had gastric bypass surgery when I weighed 255 pounds and lost 70 pounds, winding up at 185. At 5 foot 2 I am still obese, just not morbidly obese. I've weighed the same for over a year now and don't expect to lose any more, unless I exercise or diet strenuously. It was extremely difficult for me to accept that this was going to be it for me—that I was not going to lose any more. I felt like a failure, and I blamed myself. I was not exercising enough. I wasn't eating the right things. I was not disciplined enough for a rigorous diet and exercise program. Those I spoke to in my support group espoused a litany of prescriptions for success that sounded familiar—from high-protein diets to measuring what I ate to three meals a day with no snacking to Tae Bo workouts. Those suggestions were like the diet and exercise programs I'd failed at time and again before surgery. Everyone seemed to be losing much more than me. I had no desire to live on high-protein foods like meat, which didn't appeal to me. After some serious soul-searching, I concluded that I hadn't had this surgery in order to torture myself with the kind of strenuous regimens I had always avoided. I wanted to relax with food, eat what I felt like eating, and enjoy life.

Rebel that I am, I ate what I felt like eating, and eventually my weight stabilized at a high but steady 180 to 185. I got down to a size 16 or 18, which allows me to shop in a regular store. My co-morbidities have improved enormously. My diabetes is now under control with a small amount of medication instead of a huge amount. I no longer use insulin. I can do things I only dreamed about previously—including running, climbing, lifting my child, sitting on the floor and getting up, crossing my legs, fitting in a normal-size seat, walking long distances without becoming exhausted, and even ice-skating. My blood pressure and cholesterol are fine. My urinary stress incontinence is gone. I look pretty darn good, if I must say so myself. I got flooded with compliments from friends and acquaintances who are impressed with the 70-pound weight loss.

Once I began looking at the pluses, I began to see myself and the procedure as more of a success. My face, which is naturally thin, doesn't look gaunt, and my body isn't totally saggy, due to the fat I still retain. I still feel like myself at a size 18. Eating great food is one of my biggest joys. I was afraid of losing the ability to appreciate a good meal due to dumping or vomiting. I haven't. I can order an entree, eat about half, and take the rest home. If I overdo it, I dump slightly and feel tired and queasy for about twenty minutes. I love food as much as I ever did, but now I don't worry about overeating. Eventually I came to accept that I was not a failure.

I lost 50 percent of my excess weight—exactly—and Dr. Flancbaum explained to me that a 50 to 75 percent loss of excess weight is considered a SUCCESS. I'd just lost on the lower end of average. The good news is that for the first time in my life I am not GAINING. I feel great about being so much thinner and have no regrets. Like most other WLS patients, I'd do it again in a heartbeat.

HAVING REALISTIC EXPECTATIONS

Once you've had your weight loss surgery, how do you know whether it's been successful? Having realistic expectations about the results of WLS will go a long way toward avoiding disappointment with the outcome.

There was no doubt that I was most concerned with improving my health following WLS, but I also wanted to look great. There were times that I fantasized that I would be able to wear shirts that showed my midriff or tiny bikinis. I had to keep shaking myself back into reality and remember what the doctor told me—that I would be a lot less overweight, but still overweight. This surgery was going to make me healthier. And it did. It allowed me to do things I hadn't done in years, but it didn't make me thin or twenty-five years old again. In any case, now I can wear a size 14 or 16 and am delighted to say that I can shop in a regular store. Recently, my son was married, and I wore a lovely dress (not black), and people were giving me tons of compliments. For the first time in many years, I felt attractive and even a little sexy.

Hannah L., 44, 288 lbs. pre-op; 178 lbs. 3 years post-op

I feel as if WLS gave me my life back. I hated being fat, because I hated the way I looked and I hated the way I felt. But worse than that, I hated being dependent on other people. It was humiliating to ask my 75-year-old mother to do my grocery shopping for me because I got too winded to walk up and down the aisles. It was horrible to ask my teenage daughter to drive me everyplace because I could no longer fit behind the wheel of a car. Now I happily shop for my mother. I am grateful to care for my aging parent—that's my responsibility, and the way it was meant to be. I never complain about taking my daughter to soccer practice, and now I can even sit in the top of the bleachers. I'll never be really thin . . . but now I can care for myself and for those I love. I'm a person again.

Tina R., 47, 326 lbs. pre-op; 231 lbs. 5 years post-op

Before my surgery I made a list of my goals and expectations. I remember that #1 on my list was being able to sit in a chair with arms. I can do that now. Whenever I feel discouraged, I refer back to my list to remind myself how far I've come.

Jean D., 37, 347 lbs. pre-op; 219 lbs. 2½ years post-op

The goal of WLS isn't to reach your ideal weight—and very few people do. WLS takes people who are a lot overweight and makes them a lot less overweight. Surgeons consider the minimum acceptable weight loss for success to be 50 percent of excess weight. However, the majority of patients lose more, depending upon the type of procedure they have had. The lighter you are, the greater percent of excess weight you will lose. For example, consider two women, both 5 feet 4 inches tall (IBW = 120 pounds). One weighs 320 pounds and the other 270. Both then lose 100 pounds after WLS. This amount represents 50 percent of excess weight in the 320-pound woman but 75 percent in the 270-pound woman.

The exact number of pounds that will be lost is unpredictable and varies from individual to individual. In the majority of cases, the medical conditions associated with obesity will either improve or be cured. In most instances, the patient's ability to function in social, recreational, and work situations will increase. Weight loss typically slows down about a year or so after surgery and, for reasons that are not well understood, eventually reaches a plateau by 18 or 24 months. Having WLS is anything but taking the easy way out or looking for a "quick fix." Most patients have suffered from severe obesity for years and unsuccessfully tried numerous diets and treatments. Many have lost hundreds of pounds, only to regain them again and again.

WLS is the only available treatment for severe obesity that is effective long-term. For this reason, once morbidly obese people have had WLS, they have done everything they can do to lose weight and improve their health, and there is really little more they can do to change the outcome one way or another. These operations limit food intake, alter food absorption, and change energy consumption, which produces weight loss for one to two years. Thus, in my opinion, the initial weight loss achieved is due to the effects of the operation and is not so much a function of the behavior of the patient.

SURGERY ISN'T MAGIC

That said, WLS is not magic and it can be defeated. The initial period of weight loss after surgery is a "window of opportunity" for patients to make changes in their lifestyles that will promote better long-term success. For example, eating healthier, more balanced meals and exercising regularly will result in improved maintenance of weight loss. On the other hand, those who remain couch potatoes or continue to eat fatty and rich foods and "graze" on high-calorie foods during the day and into the evening will regain more weight. Although a precise formula guaranteeing success after WLS does not exist, there are simple steps that everyone should take that make sense and help promote success: eating healthier and exercising regularly.

Eat Healthier

Eating healthier after WLS is important for several reasons. Since the quantity of food that can be consumed after surgery is limited, the quality of that food becomes more critical. After WLS, patients do not have the luxury of eating "junk." They must ensure that their meals are well balanced, containing adequate amounts of protein and appropriate amounts of carbohydrate and fat. Better food choices will reduce the risk of heart disease, high blood pressure, and diabetes and help prevent weight regain.

The registered dietitian in my surgeon's office advised me to avoid snacking a lot during the day, otherwise known as grazing. Unfortunately, I've always eaten that way, and I haven't been able to really alter my lifestyle. Consequently, I've regained about 20 of the 150 pounds that I've lost. However, my weight, though high, has remained constant for about two years. How do I feel about the decision to have surgery? Great. Of course I wish I were thinner— who doesn't? But I'm far healthier than I was before. For me, the biggest perk of this whole thing is my relationship with my husband. I always feared he would lose interest in me and leave me for another woman. Although he never gave me reason to mistrust him, I could never shake the feeling. Consequently, I was clingy and moody. Our relationship (not to mention our love life) has improved vastly since I began feeling better about myself.

Janine H., 37, 356 lbs. pre-op; 226 lbs. 4 years post-op

Avoid Hunger

There have been no studies on this issue, but anecdotal evidence suggests that patients who experience the least hunger and are satisfied with the smallest amounts of food will be the most successful. Immediately after surgery, most patients lose their appetite, often for months. This is the honeymoon period when the most weight is lost. Patients become euphoric, feeling that they'll never again experience the ravenous hunger that has been their undoing. However, those appetites often return, even six or eight months later. That's when the going gets rough. If you have the impulse to snack constantly:

- Eat dense protein. If you fill up on lean meats, such as chicken or beef, you will stay full longer. Avoid crunchy carbs like chips and crackers. They go down easily and are highly caloric. Munch on low-calorie veggies, such as carrots, that fill up the pouch with fiber and stave off hunger.

- If your hunger is simply a need to keep your mouth moving, try munching on something like sunflower seeds in the shell. It takes hours to eat a whole package of 300 calories' worth.

- Reassure yourself that you probably won't be as hungry tomorrow. Many patients discover that they're constantly hungry some days and not hungry at all on others. If you overeat today, you'll probably eat less tomorrow.

- Learn to live with the sensation of hunger. It won't kill you. Many naturally thin people simply ignore hunger pangs if they arrive at an inconvenient time. The sensation will pass if you just sit with it for a while.

- Don't panic. Panic is your enemy. It will cause you to eat more. Try to be calm and remember that this is a LONG-TERM process. You didn't gain all this weight in a month, and you won't lose it that fast either.

Such dietary changes may be difficult, and patients often require professional guidance. For this reason, regular follow-up appointments and nutritional counseling are necessary. Professionally run patient-support groups can also be helpful in this regard.

Start and Stick with Your Exercise Program

Most morbidly obese people not only don't exercise—they CAN'T exercise. Trying to accomplish even everyday tasks that require physical exertion is often difficult. After surgery, however, it is advisable to try to begin an exercise regimen as soon as your surgeon permits. Mild aerobic exercises can usually be started after two or three weeks, while six to eight weeks of recovery is needed before any strength training (in order to prevent the occurrence of a hernia). Although studies indicate that exercise does not cause weight loss, it is effective in helping to keep off the pounds once they have been shed. In addition, regular exercise is healthy for your heart and cardiovascular system.

For several months after the surgery, I felt depressed. I wasn't sure if I had made the right decision. The weight was coming off and my health was improving, but I just had this vague, uneasy feeling. My therapist explained to me that it is typical to feel depressed after surgery, and that I was no longer turning to food to allay my depression. I could no longer eat a quart of Rocky Road when I felt blue. She advised me to try to find other ways to handle my feelings. Shock of shocks, I enrolled in a water-aerobics class. After working out each morning, I felt invigorated and happy. Those feelings followed me throughout the day. So, after a little bit of a rough patch, I came through and now I'm in better shape and emotionally healthier than I ever thought I would be. WLS is the best gift I ever gave myself.

John R., 34, 414 lbs. pre-op; 284 lbs. 13 months post-op

I always hated exercise. In gym class in high school I always had some excuse for not getting out and playing. It was so humiliating putting on that gym uniform that made me look like a dumpling. When I did occasionally participate, I became out of breath and felt faint—so embarrassing for a kid. As an adult, I always rationalized that I was too busy or too tired to exercise. However, since my WLS, I've decided to give it a try. I bought some cool sweat pants and a hooded sweatshirt, and every morning I walk a mile. I never thought that I would be able to go around the corner without being winded, but I've worked my way up to this, and it makes me feel great. It's a wonderful way to begin my day. Relaxing. Serene. I feel a great sense of personal accomplishment, and I think walking has helped me keep my weight stable. My eventual goal is to be able to do three miles in under an hour.

Kathy C., 43, 385 lbs. pre-op; 300 lbs. 6 months post-op

Initially, exercise will still be very difficult, until a good deal of weight has been lost. However, as time goes on it will get easier and more rewarding. Exercise can be as simple as getting out and walking—first for a quarter mile, then a half mile, and eventually working up to two miles and more. But the best exercise is doing something you enjoy. If you love it, you'll keep doing it. Most morbidly obese people have a lifetime of experience avoiding exercise, because it was painful, embarrassing, and a source of shame and failure. After surgery, exercise can be something enjoyable. Some people get high on jogging, others find hiking almost a form of worship, others might feel ecstatic while doing the polka. The trick is to find the exercise that makes you happy. Most severely obese people think of exercise as sheer pain—*fun* is not a word associated with the dreaded *E* word.

Exercise Ideas:

- Swim or do water aerobics. Swimming is gentle on the joints and less likely to cause injury.
- If you love the outdoors, walk, hike, bicycle.
- If you love people, exercise with friends. Walking alone can seem like an endless chore, but a walk with a buddy goes by very quickly.
- If you love to read, listen to a book on tape while walking or doing other exercise.
- If you love dancing, try funk-aerobics, Afro-Cuban, ballroom dancing, or country line dancing. It's a fun, easy, moderate-intensity workout and a good way to meet people.
- If you're a TV addict, set up your treadmill, stationary bicycle, or rowing machine in front of the tube and treat yourself by watching your favorite program while working out.
- Bounce on a trampoline. It's a wonderful low-impact workout and gives you the feeling of being a kid again. Put on your favorite music and jump for joy.
- Box. Boxing is a terrific stress reducer. If you can't get to a ring, do boxercise. Hang a bag and box it. Add jumping rope for more intensity.

Exercising regularly is more important than what exercise you do. Twenty minutes of aerobic exercise three times a week is effective in improving cardiovascular health. Increasing this to twenty minutes or more every day will go a long way to improving your health and maintaining your hard-earned weight loss.

The Bottom Line

The clinical course of patients after WLS is unpredictable and often characterized by physical and emotional ups and downs. The much anticipated weight loss and improvements in co-morbid conditions must frequently be balanced against episodes of nausea, food intolerance, and emotional upheaval. This is further complicated by the fact that the process of weight loss and maintenance is complex and poorly understood by medical practitioners, making precise guidance difficult.

It's the little things that have changed the most for me. People who are not severely obese cannot possibly understand what a trial everyday activities can be. Those small humiliations really eroded my self-esteem. I had trouble fitting behind the wheel of my car, tying my own shoes, or taking care of my own personal-hygiene needs (that was the WORST). I couldn't hold a child on my lap, walk half a block, or sit in a seat in a movie theater. Now that I've had the surgery, I'm still 80 pounds overweight. But do I consider it a success? You bet. I'm off insulin, and my blood pressure is normal. Beyond that—I've gotten my life back. I can do those simple things that I will never take for granted. Last night I read my granddaughter a story while she sat on my lap. What a thrill. This has not been an easy process. But I will never regret my decision. I'm a person again.

Sally G., 57, 377 lbs. pre-op; 205 lbs. 18 months post-op

I usually describe the post-operative course of patients after WLS by comparing it to pregnancy. Pregnant women can basically be divided into three groups. A small percentage of women tolerate their pregnancy very well, not experiencing any morning sickness, nausea, heartburn, etc. They essentially function normally until the time of delivery. Another small group have a miserable time with their pregnancy, manifesting frequent nausea, heartburn, extreme sensitivity to smell, and food intolerance up to the moment of delivery. The largest group has a mixture, with some nausea and morning sickness early on that improves over time. At the end of nine months, all of the women deliver, their symptoms resolve, and they are happy they did it.

Following WLS, a small number of patients have no problems. They recover uneventfully, tolerate all of their foods without difficulty, and rarely vomit. Another small group has a difficult time, experiencing a great deal of food intolerance, nausea, and vomiting. And the largest group is in between, having occasional food intolerance and nausea, but tolerating most foods. After six or nine months, most of these patients have lost a considerable amount of weight, tolerate most foods with little nausea and vomiting, and are happy with their choice.

A Personal Note

I have been performing WLS for almost ten years and have done almost 1,500 operations. By far, this has been the most emotionally and professionally satisfying aspect of my twenty-year medical career. I have witnessed hundreds of patients return to more "normal" and productive lives, usually healthier and happier than before. Many of them struggled early on, some with life-threatening complications, others with less serious ones, a few even died. But not one ever told me they regretted their decision to have WLS. I do not in any way view this as a reflection on me, as a person or a professional, but rather as a commentary on how difficult life must be for people who suffer from clinically severe obesity.

I can only hope that our understanding of obesity as a disease will continue to increase, leading to more effective treatments, and that our society's attitudes toward the obese will improve, making their lives more tolerable.

WEIGHT LOSS SURGERY FOR CHILDREN AND ADOLESCENTS

Jessica L., 17, 385 lbs. pre-op; 211 lbs. 1½ years post-op

I first learned about weight loss surgery on television. It looked like what might be an awesome solution to my problem, but I was terrified of doctors and hospitals. Needles and pills and all that stuff make me want to gag. All of that changed last year about the time of my junior prom.

Even though I was fat—and I mean hefty, over 300 pounds—I tried not to let my weight get in my way. I had friends (not boyfriends, that's for sure) and I was having a great time in high school. I was even junior-class vice president. Then it came time to start planning our prom.

I wasn't really worried about having a "date." My best friend is a boy with whom I've grown up since nursery school. He had just been dumped by his long-term girlfriend, so he promised that he'd take me. I was all set, or so I thought. The whole thing seemed so cool when I planned it out in my head. Truthfully, I have a bit of a crush on him and I thought that going to the prom together might finally make him notice me. The real problem arose when I had to find something to wear. While my girlfriends were poring over the pages of Seventeen *and* YM, *I was thinking about going to the plus-size department to find some kind of tent to put over my body. At sixteen, I was going to have to dress like the mother of the bride.*

My mom, who is also my best friend in the world, drove me to Plus Lady in the mall. I found a black strapless number in a 3XXX that looked decent on the rack. It didn't have those gross sequins that middle-aged women seem to love so much. But the shock came when I tried to zip it up and it was too tight on me. I looked like a big, fat satin balloon. Quite simply, I dissolved into tears, and I knew at that moment that I had to do something.

When we got home, I blubbered all over my mother for hours. I confessed to her that I really wanted stomach stapling but that I was terrified. I think she was pretty scared herself. I also think that she felt as if she was somehow a failure herself because I was in this situation.

We stayed up half the night talking. The next day after school, we went on-line and starting researching this surgery. Way back when, Mom was a nurse, so she understood more than me about what we were reading. But, finally, after a couple of hours on the Net, she and I both decided that this operation might be right for me.

Now it's about a year later. I had the surgery in New York City, and my doctor says I was a "trouper." I did actually barf a few times when I first got home, and the stitches really grossed me out, but it wasn't as bad as I thought.

Last night was my senior prom. I wore a dress in a size 11 junior. It was pink and shimmery and I felt like a princess. I never did get my friend to notice me, but I did get a boy named John to be my date. I think he has a little crush on me. We had a great time dancing and going to the after-prom parties. When I think about how my life has changed in one year I can't believe it.

Toni F., mother of 15-year-old WLS patient Daniel F., 274 lbs. pre-op; 156 lbs. 2 years post-op

I am one of those people in the sandwich generation. I take care of my aging parents and my growing kids. Together with working full time, I barely have time to think straight. Lots of times I let things slide. I suppose that's why I didn't realize that Daniel had a real problem for so long.

My 15-year-old son, Daniel, was always heavy. I had gestational diabetes, so he was born really big and kind of delayed in his development. As a baby, he could sit for hours playing with toys and listening to books, but he was never very active. He talked early and walked late.

When he was a kid, I didn't really encourage him to be involved in sports. Daniel always had a book in his hand. Sometimes he devoured ten books a week. How could a mother complain about a kid like that? He was smart, kind, a fantastic conversationalist, and a great cook. One of his favorite activities was reading cookbooks and then trying to duplicate some of the most elaborate recipes in them. The more ingredients and the more steps involved, the happier Daniel would be. He was particularly adept at French pastry. My fourteen-year-old son could create chocolate mousse and crème brûlée to die for. What I didn't realize was that desserts could literally have been causing Daniel to die.

I guess when it comes to our children, we can't see what we don't want to see. Daniel loved reading and being home with me, but he didn't have friends his own age. There were never teenage guests in our home and Daniel was never invited anyplace. He went to school, but he was never involved in any after-school activities. And Daniel was overweight.

Perhaps his weight was another area where I couldn't be objective. I knew that Daniel was heavy. But to me, he was just the cutest kid in the world. His engaging smile and his warm personality enabled me to focus exclusively on his inner beauty. I completely overlooked the physical.

But then Daniel started to get ill. At a regular yearly checkup, my pediatrician discovered that my son had high blood pressure. "It's not uncommon in the morbidly obese," he said so glibly. My son? Morbidly obese? There had to be some mistake. How could such a trusted family physician hurl that ugly epithet at my son? The doctor prescribed some blood-pressure medication and encouraged Daniel to exercise and lose some weight.

The next reality test arrived the following week. The nurse from the pediatrician's office called to tell me that Daniel had elevated cholesterol levels. I was shocked. Again, I went to the pharmacy and had another prescription filled.

Like a dutiful mother, I sent Daniel to a dietitian. However, they didn't really seem to hit it off. I don't think that Daniel understood why he was there. He didn't feel the gravity of the situation. As the old saying goes, You can lead a horse to water . . .

Months went by, and I tried scolding and cajoling, but nothing seemed to get Daniel off the couch except going into the kitchen. The more I scolded him, the more he ate. Then some weird symptoms started cropping up. Daniel was thirsty all the time and he was constantly urinating. After several weeks of this, I took him to the pediatrician, who referred my son to an endocrinologist. By the end of that week, Daniel was diagnosed with type II diabetes. I was shocked and guilt-ridden. Why hadn't I seen this coming? Why hadn't I been able to keep my son healthy? When we first got this awful news, I was kind of immobilized. I didn't know what to do or to whom to turn.

Then one evening, I was at my parents' house organizing my father's pills for the following week. Every Sunday afternoon I grocery shop for my parents and then do a little laundry and light housecleaning. Before I leave, I put my father's pills in a container labeled for each day of the week. As I was counting his pills, I realized that my son, my precious teenage boy, was taking more pills than my seventy-year-old father. You might call it an epiphany, but whatever it was, I realized that something needed to be done.

I cried all the way home, and as I walked through the door, I vowed that my crying days were over. I needed to help my son—I just had to figure out how. That night I sat Daniel down on his bed and talked to him about his health. He didn't appear to be concerned. But what did come pouring out were stories of ridicule he was suffering at the hands of some cruel classmates. His solace was food and his beloved novels and cookbooks. At the end of our conversation, I just sat hugging my son. Finally, he said the words I had been longing to hear: "I'm ready to take responsibility for my weight; I want to get some help." I suggested that we try yet another diet. It was then that Daniel very tentatively suggested the idea of weight loss surgery. Out of the mouths of babes.

My son had seen a segment on MSNBC about this lifesaving surgery, and he wanted to explore the option. I was terrified at the prospect. On the other hand, I knew that if his health deteriorated any further, he didn't have a very long life expectancy, something incredibly painful to admit.

After a few sleepless nights, I made a consultation with a

surgeon, and the rest is history. Daniel tolerated the operation well. He's lost about one hundred pounds so far and he's started to in-line skate. We transferred him to a new school, because when the kids at his old school heard about the operation, they teased him about that as well. In his new environment, he's making friends, reading a little less, and getting out a little more. Recently, he even had the self-confidence to ask a girl to the movies. I had to commit myself to helping Daniel make the most of his chance to lose weight. I went along with him to his postsurgical follow-ups and got good pointers on how to cook for him. A nice bonus is that I've lost a little weight myself. The best news of all, the only medication Daniel takes anymore are his vitamin pills. I feel as if I've given my son a gift by allowing him to have this operation, the gift of life.

Adam P, 16, 329 lbs. pre-op

My life in high school is pure crap. In middle school my parents got divorced, and I got myself through their fighting with double-fudge brownies and milk shakes. Before I hit the ninth grade I weighed over 200 pounds.

That's when my troubles started. Before high school I kind of faded into the background. I didn't have many friends—but nobody bothered me either. But when I gained the weight, I suddenly began getting all sorts of horrible attention. One morning when I got to my locker, there were pictures of pigs taped all over the door. You can't even imagine how humiliated I felt. Another day when I was walking down the hall, a bunch of guys made "oinking" noises at me. I don't know if I wanted to scream, punch someone, or cry. But the humiliation didn't end there. In gym class I had to change in front of the other guys into regulation gym shorts. I couldn't get them up over my thighs. As I struggled with tugging on the nylon, a group of kids circled around me and started laughing hysterically. I ran into the bathroom and threw up my guts. That only made them laugh more. I started to make excuses for why I didn't want to go to school. Stomachaches, headaches, sore throats, you name it. Anything to avoid the ridicule and torture.

A few weeks ago, my parents and I made the decision for me to have weight loss surgery. They actually agreed on something, and I *think that they'll both be there to support me. I don't know what the results will be, but I just can't wait.*

When I went to see the surgeon, he offered me a date for the operation this summer so I would not have to miss more school. I vehemently argued with him. I want this operation now! I don't want to live like this. I don't care how much school I miss or if I have to repeat the year. I just can't stand being like this.

Obesity is also a major health issue in children and adolescents. The prevalence of overweight has quadrupled, while the incidence of obesity has almost tripled over the past thirty years and continues to rise. Approximately 30 percent of children aged 6 to 11 years and adolescents aged 12 to 19 years are overweight, and 15 percent are obese. Among African-American and Hispanic children and adolescents, the prevalence of obesity is twice that among Caucasians, 24 percent compared to 12 percent. Overweight children are more likely to be obese as adults. Overweight adolescents have a 70 percent chance of becoming overweight adults, and this percentage increases to 80 percent if at least one parent is overweight.

Percentage Increase in Prevalence of Obesity in U.S. Children and Adolescents

	Children	Adolescents
1999–2000	15.3	15.5
1988–1994	11.3	10.5
1971–1974	4.0	6.2

Pediatricians, nutrition experts, and epidemiologists have bemoaned the fact that children and adolescents spend less and less time performing physical exercise and more time sitting in front of TVs, VCRs, and computers. Over 40 percent of adolescents watch more than two hours of television daily. Recommendations to alter children's diets, revamp school curricula, and encourage regular exercise have failed to stem this unhealthy tide.

Of grave concern is the accompanying increase in serious obesity-related co-morbid medical conditions, which a generation ago were primarily only adult diseases. For example, type II diabetes mellitus, which used to account for 2 to 4 percent of all childhood diabetes, has skyrocketed to almost 20 percent and is now the predominant form of childhood diabetes among African-Americans and Hispanics. Obese children are more than twelve times as likely to have high fasting blood-insulin levels, a major risk factor for type II diabetes. Hypertension, dyslipidemia, and sleep apnea occur with increased frequency among overweight and obese youth as well.

There is also an enormous social and psychological toll as these severely obese young people are subjected to ridicule and social isolation. This often results in low self-esteem and depression that translates into poor performance in school. Caucasian adolescent girls who develop a negative body image are at greater risk for developing eating disorders such as anorexia nervosa or bulimia.

Because diets, behavior modification, and exercise have been no more successful in children and adolescents than in adults, and the health risks are so high, some have proposed offering surgical therapy to appropriately selected adolescents. Unfortunately, there is little scientific data concerning weight loss surgery in adolescents. To date, only a handful of studies have been published, describing about 150 adolescents who have undergone weight loss surgery.

Adolescents who have surgery have been selected based on criteria similar to adults. In terms of weight, surgeons have utilized the same guidelines as for adults: a BMI above 40 or above 35 with serious co-morbid conditions. In terms of age, while it is difficult to determine a precise minimum age for surgical candidates, several guidelines have been employed. First, because the operation will alter eating and may potentially affect overall nutrition, there are concerns that future growth could be adversely affected. Therefore, most have adhered to the rule that the child should have reached mature bone age and stopped growing before undergoing surgery. The next issue is that of informed consent. Because weight loss surgery is a permanent procedure, the child must have a clear understanding of the procedure and what kind of commitment he or she is making. Moreover, it must be clear that the child, not the parents, wants the procedure and that there is no coercion. Similarly, because children are not totally independent, it is essential that the parents understand their critical role in their child's success. The parents must be supportive emotionally and help their child make positive lifestyle choices. They need to agree to cook appropriate meals and make sure that the child has follow-up care. For this reason, I believe that it is essential that a mental-health professional evaluate the child and the parents. Finally, the child's social environment should be analyzed for factors that could affect the success of the procedure. Is the child performing well in school and does he or she have a peer group and friends? Is the child being ridiculed? This situation often leads to a feeling of desperation on the part of the child and the parents. However, it is necessary to realize that even successful weight loss surgery may not cure all of these issues, or may even compound some of them. For example, whereas the child may have been ridiculed for eating too much and too rapidly before surgery, he or she may now be subjected to ridicule for not being able to eat certain types of food, or eat as much or as quickly. For these reasons, it is also important for a mental-health professional to remain involved, should these issues arise.

Issues related to selection notwithstanding, the results of weight loss surgery in adolescents have been excellent. Weight loss and resolution of co-morbid medical conditions have been as good as in adults. In addition, improvements in psychosocial functioning and socialization have been noteworthy. Undoubtedly, as the problem of childhood and adolescent obesity continues to increase, the role of weight loss surgery will become more clearly defined.

PAYING FOR WEIGHT LOSS SURGERY

Getting insurance coverage for WLS can be the greatest stumbling block on the way to a thinner, healthier body. "Fat discrimination" is among the few remaining socially acceptable forms of prejudice in this country, and discrimination against the obese in the insurance industry is no exception.

Polly D., 38, 238 lbs. pre-op; 144 lbs. 14 months post-op

I come from a large family. My maternal grandmother, mother, and two of my sisters are obese. I was fairly thin as a child and teenager. I was very active in high school and weighed 130 pounds when I graduated. But I began to gain weight in college. Discouraged by the way I looked, I tried Weight Watchers, Overeaters Anonymous, and the "rice diet." Each time I dieted, I lost a good deal of weight. Unfortunately, I always gained it back and then put on even more.

When I met my husband, John, I weighed 180 pounds, but he didn't seem to care about the weight. He always told me that I was beautiful. During our courtship and the early years of our marriage, my weight was stable. I was overweight but not obese, and my health was good. Then, with each pregnancy, I gained forty pounds and never lost more than ten after each birth. I started to feel that my situation was hopeless, which only caused me to find solace in food.

Raising two small children and being obese was causing stress on my body and wreaking havoc on my marriage. I developed diabetes, high cholesterol, back and knee pain, urinary stress incontinence, varicose veins, and chronic heartburn and was taking more and more medicines all the time. I was terrified that I wouldn't be around to get my kids to adulthood. My husband was constantly angry with me—blaming me for my situation. In the meantime, I made other attempts at losing weight. I even tried Optifast and fen-phen. Thankfully, I didn't have any of the adverse side effects from that drug. Again, I lost weight but put it all back on.

As the years passed, my relationship with John became nonexistent. He just couldn't handle my frequent trips to the doctor and my inability to keep up with the rest of the family on a walk or a bike ride. He was a young man and he wanted a healthy, fit wife. Several years ago, he left me.

With my self-esteem at an all-time low, I knew I needed to find a solution. It was actually my boss who told me about WLS. He broached the subject in such a caring way, I didn't feel defensive. His father had a gastric bypass and had done really well. My boss gave me the name of his dad's surgeon, and I made an appointment. Looking back, I realized that I didn't waver because I knew if I didn't do something soon, my health would continue to deteriorate and I would die.

Meeting the surgeon was an amazing experience for me. He was the first one to tell me that I wasn't solely responsible for the mess I was in. He explained that although not everything is known about the causes of obesity, clearly there are genetic and hormonal elements that play a role. I felt as if the weight (excuse the pun) of the world had been lifted from my shoulders. He explained the procedure and how it would change my life. I knew that this operation was my last chance. I had reached the end of the road.

I was so excited, and I couldn't wait to go home and tell my kids about my decision. I explained as much as I could to them. When they posed questions that I couldn't answer, I e-mailed the surgeon, who answered every one of them in detail. I knew that I was on my way to a new life.

Several days later I received a letter from my insurance company saying that they were not authorizing me to have the surgery. They claimed that obesity is not a disease and that as such they would not pay for its treatment. Never in a million years did I think that I would finally stumble upon something that could help me and now my insurance company was sabotaging me. I shored up my courage and prepared for a fight. I called the surgeon's office and they gave me direction about what I needed to do next. Since I had so many co-morbid conditions that could be helped by the surgery, including diabetes, high cholesterol, arthritis, stress incontinence, and heartburn, he told me that I should appeal the decision. My surgeon wrote a long letter, quoting the NIH and some other groups about how successful gastric bypass was for severe obesity. I also asked my internist to write a letter stating that I needed this operation to treat those diseases. He was more than happy to help me in my crusade and wrote a persuasive letter compelling them to allow me to have the operation for the sake of my health. I also wrote a letter explaining how obesity had affected me personally— how it had destroyed my health, my marriage, and made my life a living hell—and how I expected it to kill me sooner rather than later.

A few weeks later I heard from my insurance company again. This time they wanted to make sure that I had tried all other measures to lose the weight before considering surgery. They wanted a detailed diet history. I was so angry. Can you imagine them refusing someone heart surgery unless they provided a detailed record of all of their attempts to stop smoking or refrain from eating high-cholesterol foods? However, I knew I was going to have to jump through this hoop if I ever wanted to feel better. I racked my brain coming up with the details of my dieting history. I did the best I could, sent it in, and then once again waited for their answer. I called every few days asking when I would hear from them. Maybe they got tired of hearing from me, but a few weeks after my letter went out to them, I finally got a positive response. I was elated. I scheduled an appointment for my gastric bypass. Thankfully, my surgeon had a cancellation, so I was put on his schedule for the following Tuesday morning.

So far I've lost 80 pounds and I'm hoping for a little more. My diabetes was cured within six weeks and my cholesterol is normal.

My heartburn and stress incontinence were also gone within a few weeks. The only pills I take now are vitamins and an iron supplement. Best of all, my boss who recommended this surgery to me visited me every day while I was recuperating—bringing me flowers, cards, and little gifts. It took me a while to realize that he was interested in me—fat or thin. We've been dating for about nine months, and my future is looking pretty bright.

Insurers need to be convinced that obesity is a disease and be persuaded to pay for its treatment as they do other conditions, regardless of whether people's eating habits contribute to their obesity. Tobacco, alcohol and drug use, accidental trauma, violence, and HIV/AIDS account for the vast majority of preventable deaths in the U.S. and a significant percentage of health-care expenditures. Yet no insurer would dare deny treatment for lung cancer, coronary heart disease, stroke, hepatitis, or HIV/AIDS based upon the notion that the illness was, in part, self-induced.

This is especially true of the federal government, which is the nation's largest insurer by virtue of the Medicare and Medicaid programs. At present, obesity is not considered a disease according to the Medicare Coverage Manual, and therefore treatment of obesity is not a covered benefit:

> *Obesity itself cannot be considered an illness. The immediate cause is a caloric intake which is persistently higher than caloric output.*
>
> *Program payment may not be made for treatment of obesity alone since this treatment is not reasonable and necessary for the diagnosis or treatment of an illness or injury.*

On the other hand, Medicare can cover WLS on a limited basis:

> *However, although obesity is not in itself an illness, it may be caused by illnesses such as hypothyroidism, Cushing's disease, and hypothalamic lesions [glandular disorders]. In addition, obesity can aggravate a number of cardiac and respiratory diseases as well as diabetes and hypertension. Therefore, services*

in connection with the treatment of obesity are covered when such services are an integral and necessary part of a course of treatment for one of these illnesses.

. . . [G]astric bypass surgery . . . is performed for patients with extreme obesity. Gastric bypass surgery for extreme obesity is covered under the program if:

1. *It is medically appropriate for the individual to have such surgery.*
2. *The surgery is to correct an illness, which caused the obesity or was aggravated by the obesity.*

Such limited coverage by Medicare is inconsistent with other services and treatments for which Medicare does provide coverage, such as inpatient and outpatient alcohol and drug detoxification and rehabilitation, including antismoking drugs. Medicare and other insurance carriers frequently cover treatment of sexual dysfunction or infertility, neither of which addresses life-threatening ailments, while completely excluding any and all treatment for obesity, including surgery. Some insurers require so much documentation that meeting the requirements is much like rolling a stone up a mountain.

Ironically, making it difficult for people to have WLS actually increases the costs to insurance companies by denying enrollees lifesaving surgery. For example, a person with diabetes will spend thousands of insurance dollars on medications and the treatment of complications, including such expensive procedures as coronary bypass or peripheral vascular surgery, hemodialysis, or a kidney transplant. It would be cost-effective in the long run to pay for one surgical procedure, like a gastric bypass, and eliminate the need for other long-term expenses. However, insurance companies don't view subscribers as long-term responsibilities. Instead, they gamble that their customers will likely change carriers before they can recoup their investment.

Nevertheless, there are some indications that the insurance-coverage situation is improving and will continue to do so as time goes on. The recognition of obesity as a dire national-health problem will eventually cause insurers to cover treatment for it, and legislative initiatives to regulate HMO abuses will also help. The American Obesity Association (www.obesity.org), a patient and professional advocacy group, and many professional organizations involved in the treatment of obesity are actively lobbying Congress and state legislatures to amend their codes and recognize obesity as a disease. Legislation requiring health-insurance coverage for weight loss programs has recently been passed by the state of Indiana and is under consideration in several others, including Georgia, Hawaii, Maryland, Michigan, Montana, and Virginia. Until similar laws are enacted in all states, patients will need information about how to fight their insurers for coverage.

The American Obesity Association has published a guidebook entitled *Weight Management and Health Insurance,* which offers suggestions on obtaining reimbursement for obesity treatment. Numerous published studies documenting the increased cost associated with obesity and the health and economic benefits of long-term weight loss are turning the tide. During the past few years, for example, United Healthcare, which used to have a blanket exclusion for the treatment of obesity in most of its policies, reversed its decision and now covers WLS. In my practice in New York City, over 90 percent of patients that I have evaluated have received approval for surgery by their insurance company.

GETTING APPROVAL FOR SURGERY

A brief review of the ABCs of current insurance lingo is useful when trying to obtain insurance approval for WLS. "Traditional" or "indemnity" plans allow enrollees to select doctors of their choice and the carrier and patient each pay a percentage of the fee, usually 80 percent/20 percent or 70 percent/30 percent. Indemnity policies are becoming increasingly rare but offer the most latitude. Patients who hold these policies are usually not required to have a primary-care physician (PCP) or obtain a referral to see a specialist. Preferred Provider Organizations (PPO) or Point of Service (POS) plans also offer a fair number of choices in terms of physicians. These plans may or may not require the approval of a PCP before seeing a specialist. Also, patients who subscribe to a PPO or POS can usually see a physician out-of-network if they are willing to pay a greater portion of the charges. Health Maintenance Organizations (HMO) or Managed Care Organizations (MCO) are the most restrictive. HMOs usually require patients to have a PCP and obtain his or her approval before seeing a specialist, and often mandate that patients see only physicians who are participants in their provider networks.

Many patients with severe obesity receive Medicare (usually as SSI Disability) or Medicaid, which operate differently. Medicare is a federal program and thus is governed by federal law. At this time, Medicare does not recognize obesity as a disease and therefore does not pay for obesity treatment, including the treatment of morbid obesity. However, Medicare will pay for WLS to treat a complication of obesity that will benefit from weight loss, such as severe arthritis, sleep apnea, etc. Unfortunately, because Medicare does not preapprove treatments or procedures, it is impossible to find out ahead of time whether a given patient's WLS will be covered. As a rule, I insist that Medicare beneficiaries have at least two letters recommending WLS from treating physicians before surgery in the event that Medicare denies coverage after the fact and an appeal is necessary.

Medicaid is also a federal program; however, it is administered by each state. Each jurisdiction makes its own rules and determinations about coverage. Some states cover WLS, such as New York, New Jersey, Massachusetts, Pennsylvania, Virginia, and California, while others, such as Ohio, do not. Each state also has its own requirements regarding documentation and approval. Because insurance companies are often reluctant to cover WLS, getting approval for this treatment is more complicated than for other types of medical care. A simple phone call will not suffice as it does for gallbladder, hernia, breast, or cancer surgery. Most insurance carriers have specific requirements for patients seeking WLS, and the decision is often made by a medical director, not a claims adjuster. Therefore, a letter of medical necessity justifying the procedure is needed.

Both your surgeon and your PCP should write letters to your insurance company explaining that you need the surgery and why. If you are enrolled in an HMO, your PCP's letter may be the more important, because he or she is the "gatekeeper." In addition, the HMO will likely view your PCP as objective and is more likely to listen to him or her than to a surgeon whom they see as having a vested interest in performing the operation. Therefore, it is necessary to seek a PCP who is sympathetic to your special needs and problems as someone with severe obesity and is willing to act as an advocate in your quest for surgery. Even so, the PCP may want you to exhaust other approaches like dieting and drugs first. Agree to whatever your PCP recommends, but keep going back every month to be weighed and keep detailed records of each visit and your progress.

Your surgeon must be willing to support you in your quest for coverage, including writing a convincing letter on your behalf. His or her staff should be diligent in following up with phone calls and supplying the required information. Many bariatric practices have extensive experience dealing with insurance companies and are quite expert at gaining approvals. The following is a sample of the letter I write to insurance companies.

Note: It is critical that the letter clearly state that the disease for which treatment is being sought is Morbid Obesity (ICD-9 code 278.01). Because morbid obesity has its own International Classification of Disease code, it is considered to be a different disease from obesity (ICD-9 code 278.0).

TO: Insurance Carrier
       Address
RE: Name:
       Policyholder:
       Certificate/ID #   Group#

Preauthorization for Surgery (Name of Operation, CPT code)

To whom it may concern:
This letter is regarding XXX, who was evaluated at St. Luke's–Roosevelt Center for weight loss surgery. The Center is composed of a multidisciplinary group of health-care providers, including general

surgeons, internists, nutritionists/dietitians, and behaviorists, who have special interest and expertise in the treatment of obesity and its associated co-morbid conditions.

Our pre-operative surgical evaluation consists of a complete history and physical examination, baseline laboratory studies to screen for and evaluate co-morbid conditions, a consultation with a registered dietitian, and, if clinically indicated, an evaluation by a licensed mental-health professional.

Our findings are as follows: Mr./Ms. XXX is a XX-year-old who weighs XXX lbs. and is XX inches tall, corresponding to a Body Mass Index of XX Kg/m^2. He/she suffers from morbid obesity (278.01) complicated by the following obesity-related co-morbid conditions:

1)   5)
2)   6)
3)   7)
4)   8)

Results of our dietary and psychological screening have shown that the patient has failed dietary treatments in the past and no psychological problems were identified that, in our opinion, would preclude or contraindicate surgical treatment.

Based upon the degree of obesity and the associated conditions described above, we feel that this patient is an appropriate candidate for Name of Operation (CPT code XXXXX).

A lengthy discussion was held with the patient describing the procedure, including the indications, complications, risks, benefits, and the necessity for long-term follow-up care. This surgery is necessary to reduce weight and, thereby, achieve improvement or resolution of the above-mentioned co-morbid conditions. Surgical treatment is only considered for those patients with a BMI greater than 40 Kg/m^2 (100 lbs. above ideal body weight) or in patients with a BMI greater than 35 Kg/m^2 with especially serious co-morbid conditions. These guidelines are in accordance with the recommendations of the NIH Consensus Development Conference Statement (1991), Clinical Guidelines (1998), and the Practical Guide (2000), the American Obesity Association/Shape Up America! (1997), the American Heart Association (1997), and the World Health Organization (1998). This surgery is not cosmetic surgery but rather lifesaving surgery. Long-term results following surgical treatment have been documented to be excellent, with most patients achieving a weight loss of at least half of their excess body weight and improvements in or resolution of many of their obesity-related, co-morbid conditions.

Surgery is scheduled for XXXXX. [A date is mandatory.] We appreciate your consideration and request precertification and approval of our recommendations and making available this treatment, which can extend the quantity of life, improve the quality of life, and decrease the cost of health care for this patient. If you have any questions, please feel free to contact us. We await your response.

Sincerely,

The initial request for preauthorization may be approved, returned for additional information, or denied. Many insurance programs use their own criteria for WLS, which differ from or are more detailed than those proposed by the NIH, AOA, and WHO. Some examples of such criteria are higher BMIs (above 45), the presence of certain co-morbidities (diabetes, hypertension, coronary artery disease, sleep apnea), failure of medically supervised diets for specific lengths of time (12 or 18 months), and a formal psychological screening. For these reasons, it is important to:

- *Document your weight reduction programs.* Your insurance carrier may require you to document that you have made serious attempts to lose weight without surgery, preferably in medically supervised weight reduction programs. Put together a detailed diet history listing every weight loss program you have ever undertaken, including the dates, amounts lost and regained, and the name of the dietitian or physician who supervised them. If you don't remember all of your attempts at losing weight, make educated guesses. If you can obtain documentation directly from the program or supervisor, do so.
- *Seek medical help early and repeatedly for all weight-related complaints.* You want to have all your co-morbidities documented thoroughly, even seemingly minor ones. If

your joints ache, or you have urinary stress incontinence or heartburn, miss menstrual periods, get out of breath walking up stairs, snore, or have swollen ankles, go to the doctor for treatment. Keep visiting your doctor regularly and mention each complaint at every visit. If you are morbidly obese but otherwise relatively healthy, you may have a harder time with certain carriers, despite the fact that a BMI > 40 is an independent risk factor for other complications and death. Even though it makes sense to operate before serious problems arise, the insurance companies don't necessarily see it that way. Two out of three morbidly obese people have co-morbid conditions, so you need to be aware of your body and the kinds of problems you have that normal-weight people don't have. These can include psychological problems such as depression and anxiety due to your weight.

- *Make sure your complaints are accurately documented in your chart.* If you have joint pain, urinary stress incontinence, heartburn, shortness of breath after mild activity, amenorrhea, difficulty sleeping, make sure they are noted in your chart. Get all the tests you need to document these co-morbidities and save all of your prescriptions for the treatment of obesity-related problems. If your PCP is not being helpful in this regard, you may need to find someone more sympathetic.

DENIAL AND APPEAL

In the event the request for preauthorization is denied, all policies offer a mechanism by which the decision can be appealed. The best strategy for the appeal will depend upon the specific terms of your policy.

What to Do if Your Policy Has an Exclusion for Obesity Treatment

Many insurance policies have exclusions for certain conditions, such as obesity, which means that they are not obligated to cover treatment of that condition. Some policies exclude only dietary or drug treatment for obesity, while others have total exclusions, which apply to *all* forms of obesity treatment, including surgery.

The first thing to do if your policy has such an exclusion is to check the exact wording. Often the exclusion is for the treatment of obesity, not *morbid obesity*. Morbid obesity is considered to be a separate disease from obesity, according to the International Classification of Diseases, with an ICD-9 code 278.01; obesity is ICD-9 code 278.0. The significance of this distinction cannot be overemphasized, because a policy that excludes treatment of obesity may be obligated to cover the treatment of morbid obesity.

If your policy has a total exclusion, your options are limited. If the exclusion is well written and ironclad, it will be very difficult to contest their denial, since the whole basis of your health coverage is contractual. If your insurance company doesn't promise treatment for obesity, then you can't get it. Most people miss out because they don't realize that the exclusions aren't usually all that clear. Insurance companies don't want to make exclusions clear, so they make them nebulous, using terms like *experimental* or *not medically necessary*. These can frequently be fought and won.

If your policy contains an ironclad exclusion, consider alternatives. The best option in this circumstance may be to change policies if you have the opportunity. Wait until the time for open enrollment comes and make the switch to a more favorable insurer. If you are currently enrolled in an HMO, consider joining a plan with more freedom of choice, such as a POS or PPO. Do not automatically give up if your policy contains an exclusion. If you have insurance through your employer or a union, speak to the human-resources director. Your employer may not even be aware of the existence of the exclusion or its ramifications. If you are a government employee, contact a lawyer, the attorney general, or a patient's rights organization for help. You may be able to convince someone that it is improper for the government to offer health insurance that excludes treatment of a disease that afflicts over one-half of the population.

The other factor working to the benefit of insurance companies is intimidation. When a patient gets a letter with a corporate letterhead definitively stating that such-and-such procedure is not covered, the normal human response is to say—that's it, there's no hope. People automatically assume that there is no chance of being covered. The reality is that the insurance companies all have an appeals process, and you can use that process to your advantage. If your initial request is turned down, the carrier is legally obligated to tell you what your appeal rights are. Generally, you have 30 to 60 days to file an appeal, with whatever new information you have.

What to Do in Order to Win

Remember That You Are in the Right: The National Institutes of Health, World Health Organization, and the American Obesity Association/Shape Up America! have each published guidelines for treatment of obesity that include WLS for the most severely obese individuals. WLS is not experimental or radical. It is the most effective form of treatment available for morbid obesity and the only treatment that consistently results in significant long-term weight loss.

You Are Your Own Best Advocate: Your PCP and surgeon may be sympathetic and want to be helpful, but they are also busy caring for other patients. Their office staffs will not have time and motivation to continuously advocate for you. You must be willing and ready to assist them and even take the lead. This may involve tracking down information and old medical records in addition to making frequent, repetitive phone calls and writing numerous letters.

See Yourself as a Customer: Remember that you pay for your insurance; it's not free. Therefore you need to insist on receiving the services you need.

Accept That Winning Is Not Going to Be Easy: Insurance carriers are large, impersonal, and seemingly invincible organizations. You may experience frustration and disappointment trying to overcome their extensive bureaucracy. Be prepared to spend hours on paperwork and research, money on phone calls, faxes, and copying, and possibly hiring a lawyer.

Be Persistent. Don't Back Off at the First Sign of Resistance: This process is one example where "the squeaky wheel gets the grease." Insurance companies come up with all sorts of excuses all the time, such as "this was a preexisting condition so we're not covering it—ever." Be persistent and let them know you do not intend to let them get away with that. A preexisting condition has to have a time frame and can't be denied permanently. Be persistent so the insurance company will decide it's not worth the trouble to deal with you and give you what you want to make you go away. One patient got approval by faxing and e-mailing her insurer supporting documentation every day. Each time she faxed a letter she called to see if they received it. (Be sure to use their toll-free numbers for these communications.) Her repeated phone calls tied up valuable employee time. She faxed so many times they accused her of tying up their fax machine. "I basically drove them nuts," she recalls, but she got her approval.

Enlist Your Employer's Help: One thing that may be in your favor is that you probably have your insurance through either your or your spouse's employer. Instead of being secretive about having WLS, try to bring your employer in on your plans if the insurance company gives you a hard time. Go to the company's insurance liaison or human-resources department—each company has one—and explain that you would be a more productive worker if you lost weight. Employers don't like paying workman's compensation or disability. Your employer can take their business elsewhere. The bigger the company, the more clout it has. For instance, ten years ago specific changes were made to the plan Santa Clara County, California, had with Kaiser Permanente, because Santa Clara insisted on them. Also, many corporations may be unaware that their plan is denying necessary medical treatment to a significant number of their employees.

Document, Document, Document: Keep meticulous records, including as much detail as possible. Write down every contact you have with everyone from the insurance carrier—detailing the date, time, person spoken to, and what was said. Insurance-company employees often contradict themselves, and you want to be in the position of saying, "But on March 3, Mrs. Smith, your benefits analyst, told me you do not specifically exclude my particular condition."

Contact Everyone You Can Think of, and Copy Them at the End of Every Letter to Your Insurance Company: Enlist your local, state, and federal legislators in your fight. Many politicians like to help constituents with problems and are actively involved in the effort to make health insurers more responsive to the public. Insurers do not like mail from government officials or licensing departments. These require responses, which makes more work for them. If all else fails, consider contacting the media. If your case is particularly heartrending or you have been treated heartlessly by the insurance company, you may get coverage by a local news station or newspaper, especially in these days of rising political pressure on managed care.

Provide Back-up Documentation: Include as much documentation as possible with your appeal. Include information from your doctor about your medical condition; documentation from experts about how surgery is the only cure for morbid obesity; your diet history; information from support groups and the Internet; the opinion of another, uninvolved doctor or surgeon; your own testimony about living with the pain of obesity. Insurance companies are often persuaded by the weight of evidence. The more letters you include the better. Include statements supporting WLS from all of the medical organizations and experts who have come out in favor of it. A number of statements from major health-care organizations endorsing surgical treatment of obesity that can be used in your letter are summarized below.

STATEMENTS ENDORSING SURGICAL TREATMENT OF OBESITY

National Institutes of Health Consensus Development Conference (1991)

> The surgical procedures currently in use [such as Roux-en-Y gastric bypass and vertical banded gastroplasty] are capable of inducing significant weight loss in severely obese patients, which in turn has been associated with amelioration of most of the co-morbid conditions that have been studied . . . while limited success has been achieved by a variety of

techniques that include medically supervised weight loss and intensive behavior modification . . . a major drawback of the nonsurgical approach is failure to maintain reduced body weight in the vast majority of patients.

Shape Up America!/American Obesity Association: Guidances for the Treatment of Adult Obesity (1996)

Surgical treatment for obesity should be considered for patients with a BMI above 40 or a BMI above 35 with co-morbidities or other risk factors.

American Heart Association Science Advisory and Coordinating Committee: Obesity and Heart Disease (1997)

When the BMI is above 35 and co-morbidities exist, gastrointestinal surgery becomes a consideration. When the BMI is above 40, surgery is the treatment of choice. The experience of the surgeon and type of operation chosen predict outcome. In general, a Roux-en-Y gastric bypass is superior to gastric plication [gastroplasty].

American Dietetic Association: Position Paper on Weight Management (1997)

Surgical treatment of obesity should be limited to patients with a BMI over 40 or BMI over 35 and severe co-morbid conditions related to the obesity. Roux-en-Y gastric bypass and vertical banded gastroplasty are the most commonly performed and widely accepted procedures currently in use . . .

Seventy percent of patients maintain a loss of 50 percent of their initial excess weight for 5 years. Improvements in cardiovascular functioning, lipid profile, sleep apnea, physical activity, and work abilities have been reported.

World Health Organization: Obesity: Preventing and Managing the Global Epidemic (1998)

Surgery is now considered to be the *most effective* way of reducing weight, and maintaining weight loss, in severely (BMI over 35) and very severely obese (BMI over 40) subjects. On a kg/weight loss basis, surgical treatment has been estimated after four years to be less expensive than any other treatment.

NIH, National Heart Lung and Blood Institute: Clinical Guidelines on the Identification, Evaluation, and Treatment of Overweight and Obesity in Adults—The Evidence Report (1998)
Gastrointestinal surgery (gastric restriction [vertical gastric banding] or gastric bypass [Roux-en-Y]) can result in substantial weight loss, and therefore is an available weight loss option for well-informed and motivated patients with BMI over 40 or BMI over 35, who have co-morbid conditions and acceptable operative risks.

NIH, National Heart Lung and Blood Institute, North American Association for the Study of Obesity: The Practical Guide— Identification, Evaluation, and Treatment of Overweight and Obesity in Adults (2000)
Weight loss surgery provides medically significant sustained weight loss for more than 5 years in most patients. Surgery is an option for well-informed and motivated patients who have clinically severe obesity (BMI > 40) or a BMI > 35 and serious co-morbid conditions.

The Letter of Appeal

A thoughtful, well-written letter of appeal can go a long way toward convincing an insurance company that your WLS should be covered. In addition to a letter from you, letters of appeal should also be submitted by your surgeon and your PCP. Insurance companies want you to go away without a fight. If they see you're ready to put up an effective battle, they may just cave in.

TO: Insurance Carrier
      Address

RE: Name:
      Policyholder:
      Certificate/ID #   Group#

Appeal of Denial for Surgery (Name of Operation, CPT code)

Dear XXX [it is best to identify a specific person]:

I am writing to appeal your denial of the request by the above-noted patient for weight loss surgery (Name of Operation, CPT code____).

Mr./Ms. XXX is a XX-year-old who weighs XXX lbs. and is XX inches tall, corresponding to a Body Mass Index of XX Kg/m². Based upon ALL currently accepted medical criteria, he/she suffers from morbid obesity (278.01). Morbid obesity is a life-threatening disease that currently afflicts over 10 million American adults. It is associated with premature death and numerous medical conditions including: diabetes, hypertension, hyperlipidemia, coronary artery disease and stroke, several forms of cancer, obstructive sleep apnea, arthritis, gout, gallstones, GERD, menstrual irregularity, infertility, and depression. Many activities of daily living are also affected, such as washing, bathing, and dressing.

Mr./Ms. XXX suffers from the following obesity-related co-morbid conditions:

1)   5)
2)   6)
3)   7)
4)   8)

Mr./Ms. XXX has been thoroughly evaluated and, in my professional judgment, is an appropriate candidate for this treatment. In addition, he/she has tried numerous other approaches for weight loss, including XXX [examples: Weight Watchers, Jenny Craig, Atkins Diet, Zone Diet, behavior modification, etc.], without success.

Numerous organizations, including the NIH [Consensus Development Conference Statement (1991), Clinical Guidelines (1998), and Practical Guide (2000)], the American Obesity Association/Shape Up America! (1996), and the World Health Organization (1998), have endorsed surgical treatment for this degree of obesity. Surgical treatment is only considered for those patients with a BMI greater than 40 Kg/m²(100 lbs. above ideal body weight) or patients with a BMI greater than 35 Kg/m² with especially serious co-morbid conditions. This surgery is not cosmetic surgery but rather lifesaving surgery. Long-term results following surgical treatment have been excellent, with most patients achieving a weight loss of at least half of their excess body weight and improvements in or resolution of many of their obesity-related, co-morbid conditions. Studies have also demonstrated surgical treatment of obesity to be cost-effective, reducing overall health costs and allowing many people to return to work.

I strongly urge you to reconsider your decision and make available this treatment, which can extend the quantity of life, improve the quality of life, and decrease the cost of health care for this patient. If you have any questions, please feel free to contact me.

Sincerely

Your Doctor, M.D.

With this letter, I enclose a copy of the original request, the letter of denial, copies of the statements detailed on pages 167–169, as well as the American Obesity Association's statement on Obesity Surgery (included in Appendix A). Copies should be sent to as many appropriate individuals as one can identify.

You, as the person suffering from morbid obesity, can and should write an appeal letter of your own. A personal plea can be very effective. Include a personal account of your lifelong battle with obesity, how it has affected your health, your lifestyle, your career and social choices, and other aspects of your life. Outline your family history of obesity, the diets you have tried and failed, and the problems you expect to arise in the future. Make it clear that if your surgery is denied, you will seek help from your local legislators and the media.

Consulting an Attorney

Although many people successfully win appeals on their own, you might need to consult with an attorney. Start with your city's bar association, which is most knowledgeable about the expertise of local attorneys. Failing that, try your state's bar association. If you receive your health insurance through work, you will do best to ask for a lawyer with experience in ERISA (Employee Retirement Income Security Act). ERISA is a federal law that governs employer-provided pension benefits, which include health insurance. The original intent of ERISA was to stem abuses in union pension plans, but following the doctrine of unintended consequences, it evolved into a statute that prevents patients from suing their HMOs. A change in this statute is high on the legislative agendas of both parties, but (as of this writing) has not yet been passed. Once patients have the right to sue for punitive damages if death or injury occur as a result of an insurance denial, coverage for obesity surgery will probably become much easier to obtain. Lawyers knowledgeable about ERISA are most likely to be familiar with the whole issue of denials of health-care coverage and will know how to best fight and win your case. You should be aware that 95 percent of lawsuits never go to trial. They're either resolved by a summary judgment, where the court looks at the evidence and makes a decision, or settled out of court by the parties.

Government employees, including city, county, and state workers, are NOT covered by ERISA. Therefore, they or their heirs CAN sue an insurance company for punitive damages if someone dies or is injured as a result of the denial of treatment for their obesity. This provides some extra leverage for government workers.

When selecting an attorney, some useful questions to ask are: How many appeals have you fought? How many have you won? Have you represented any clients trying to get this type of surgery? Do you know what my insurance company's history is when it comes to this type of denial? It may be preferable to seek an attorney who will work for a fixed fee or on a contingency basis; paying an hourly fee can quickly become very expensive.

There are two on-line lists that assist people with obesity-surgery insurance problems—OSSGinsurance@onelist.com and OSSG-helponinsurance@egroups.com—in addition to the American Obesity Association: www.obesity.org.

17

LOST: 180 POUNDS GAINED: HEALTH AND EIGHT POUNDS OF BABY

Denise Rasley, 26, 348 lbs. pre-op; 168 lbs. 2 years post-op

I don't remember a time when I wasn't overweight. I started a lifetime of dieting at six and since then I've been on every diet known to man. By junior high, I was known as "beluga." I remember once my grandmother tried to get me to lose weight by paying me a dollar a pound. She actually paid me $25 when I got down to 175 from 200.

I went away to college at 175 pounds and gained the freshman 15. Then I got hit with a terrible disease—polycystic ovary syndrome—which is associated with a hormone imbalance that causes you to gain weight. They're not sure if it's the weight that causes the polycystic ovaries, or the hormone imbalance that causes you to gain weight. Whichever it was, I stopped getting my period—although I still got terrible cramps—and I started packing on the pounds. It's a vicious cycle. Once you have polycystic ovaries you can't take weight off easily. And the more weight you gain the worse the polycystic ovaries get. I wound up infertile and insulin resistant.

I never thought I was going to marry or have a child, but meeting Dave changed all that. We lived hundreds of miles apart and met at an Internet gamers convention. We spent two weeks together, went back to our separate cities, and he proposed six weeks later. It sounds fairy-tale-ish, but in a way that's what it was. A lot of little girls grow up and want the fairy tale. I didn't want the *fairy tale until I met the prince. When we got married everything seemed to click. I wanted to raise a child with him more than anything else in the world. He loved me unconditionally. No one but my parents had ever loved me that way before. There was so much love I wanted to share it with a child, but my weight was a major obstacle. I wasn't ovulating, due to the polycystic-ovary disease. By the time we got married I weighed 290 pounds, and then I just kept gaining. They put me on Redux and I gained weight—on a 1,200-calorie-a-day diet. My doctor swore I was cheating, but actually I was eating less than the 1,200 calories a day. We tried to get pregnant for two years. I took Clomid, which gave me mood swings and didn't make me ovulate. We did intrauterine insemination, charting, checking, etc. It wasn't working. My fertility specialist said that unless I lost the weight I probably would never get pregnant, unless we used in vitro fertilization, which we couldn't afford. By this time I weighed 348 pounds, so I wasn't really healthy enough to carry to term anyway.*

I had always been the type of person who was skeptical about weight loss surgery. I didn't believe you should mutilate your body just to lose weight. I figured I was happily married, had a decent job, so why not just accept myself the way I was. But, on the other hand, I couldn't walk to the end of my driveway without severe shin-splints. I was out of breath from any exertion. My hands and feet were swollen and I sweated constantly. Standing for any length of time hurt. I couldn't find decent clothes to wear. I had to run to the rest room every hour because of pressure on my bladder. My back hurt constantly. And every time a commercial for weight loss surgery at a nearby bariatric program came on the radio, I burst into tears. I even got depressed going to Cedar Point, the local amusement park, because I'm a roller-coaster fanatic and I could only fit on the merry-go-round. I hated the way I was living. Actually, I didn't feel I was living—I felt I was sitting on the sidelines watching life go by.

I decided to have surgery in 1998. I started researching it on the Internet, which was a very big help to me. I found out that it's no longer called stomach stapling—that the most popular and successful operation today is gastric bypass. My parents were very supportive, but Dave was terrified. He had a friend who'd had weight loss surgery—the old stomach stapling, not gastric bypass—and she popped the staples, had blood clots, and couldn't keep anything down. It didn't matter to Dave if I was fat or thin. He just wanted me to be alive and happy. Eventually, though, he was convinced that I'd done enough research to make sure it was safe.

How was the surgery? I went into it resigned. The day before, we had to get up at four A.M. to drive to the hospital. I thought I was going to be terrified, but I slept all the way there. I even fell asleep in my room before surgery and afterward in the recovery room. It was one of the best decisions I've ever made in my life. I was so relaxed, until they made me walk just four hours after surgery. I hated those nurses. They got me up every four hours after that. As much as I complained at the time, I was kind of glad because then I had no excuse not to walk when I got home. Surgery was the easy part. The hard part was watching food commercials at home. I wanted all that food, even though I wasn't hungry. I was living on chicken broth. I was on clear foods and purees for four weeks, at six weeks soft foods, but after week seven I could eat anything.

After surgery it was like I started my life all over again. For the first time in as long as I could remember, I wasn't physically hungry. I didn't have the need or desire to eat. Let's face it, everything in this country revolves around food. Weddings, funerals, parties. Sometime when I was growing up I started becoming hungry all the time. I could eat and then an hour later I'd be hungry again. My body didn't work right. I'm not sure if it was because of the polycystic ovaries or because I was always being put on diets so I constantly craved "forbidden" foods like cake and cookies. For the first six to twelve weeks after surgery, I had to be reminded to eat.

Now when it comes to food, I don't feel the least bit deprived. I feel more alive and gifted than before. People go out to eat with me and they're amazed. They think all I can eat is two bites and I'm done. But I can eat salad, filet mignon, even a little dessert, just not a restaurant-size portion. I eat a suggested serving size of whatever I want. After surgery I mourned a little because I couldn't eat huge portions, but I soon realized that the food I do eat tastes better than I ever remember. Things I used to love—like greasy, dripping french fries and onion rings—aren't appealing anymore. With food that is appealing, the texture, variety, and experience of eating is now a joy.

It wasn't all easy. I had to get used to being upset, to being angry, to allowing myself to feel. There were times I'd burst into tears or scream or holler and not know why I was doing it—but it was because I was allowing myself to feel something that I'd hidden before with what I was eating. I still eat emotionally sometimes, but I don't have the same drive to overeat that I had before. My stomach is reduced to the size where I can listen to its signals. I'm now more in touch with my body. I also don't punish myself anymore if I eat something unhealthy or sweet. If I eat too much sugar my body punishes me, but I've learned my limits. Too much ice cream one night had me throwing up, then falling asleep, then having diarrhea the next day. I didn't make a conscious decision to change my eating habits—I learned that if I ate too much or too fast, I'd get sick, so I started listening to my body.

My life changed radically in many other ways. I lost 180 pounds in one year. People I knew didn't recognize me when they saw me, which was extremely disorienting. I'd look in the mirror and I didn't recognize myself. I went through several wardrobes. Everything made me cry. When we went to Wal-Mart and I fit into a misses size for the first time, I cried. That same night we went to dinner and I couldn't eat what was set in front of me and I cried. I went to Cedar Point amusement park and rode every single ride in the park and I cried. I called my mom and said, "I did it. I'm living again."

People started treating me differently. I worked at a TV station for a while but was laid off two weeks after surgery. Six months later I went back to visit. People who wouldn't talk to me while I worked there fell all over themselves to compliment me. Other people who only talked about me now refused to say a word, because they couldn't put me down anymore. I went from being considered lazy and someone who didn't take care of herself to being considered admirable, a hard worker. Meanwhile, I was the same person. I'd just gotten a physical problem corrected.

With time my personality changed. I'm more outgoing now and less likely to put up with people's put-downs. My sense of self-worth has gone through the roof. Before I had surgery, I was always trying to please other people. I felt that if I pleased them they'd like me. If they liked me, they'd overlook the fact that I was fat. Now my attitude is—if you don't like me you're not worth my time. My relationships have changed—for the better—because, with the world not treating me so rudely, I'm a lot more pleasant to be around and I'm a lot more self-assured. There are people I decided I don't need—people who only wanted me around because I was a convenient kicking post. There are also people who suddenly wanted to be friends after I lost weight. I don't need them either. I even quit a job I hated to go back to school to become an English teacher. And I'm working with a legislator in Ohio to change the laws so that obese people can get health-care coverage for weight loss surgery.

I don't miss being fat. I was a little fearful of becoming thin, because I was always the fat, smart one. I wondered if I suddenly wasn't fat, would I still be considered smart? It sounds stupid, but being normal can be scary. There's nothing to set you apart. As much as we don't want to stand out because we're the biggest one in the room, it's also scary to blend in. I wondered if I was normal, would there be anything unique about me? Would my personality still be the same, would the people who liked me still like me? There's a lot of fear and self-doubt. It's one of the emotional aspects of weight loss that people don't consider.

Of course the absolutely best moment since I had surgery was the moment that I found out I was pregnant. Women are not supposed to get pregnant until at least a year after the surgery, because it's dangerous to lose weight during pregnancy. I followed instructions, and a year after surgery I stopped using contraception. Then I went to my family doctor and told him I was a week late for my period. They took a pee cup and I sat there for five minutes, ready to head out the door. For three years I'd been disappointed, one pregnancy test after another. I figured it wasn't going to happen this time either, so I might as well leave. Before I got my coat on, the nurse came in the room and said, "I have a question for you." I said, "You might as well tell me I'm not pregnant; I know that." Then she asked, "I want to know why you lost all this weight just to gain some of it back. You're going to gain at least twenty to thirty pounds over the next nine months." I started screaming so loud that one of the doctors came in and asked if I needed a tranquilizer. That had to be the best moment of my life.

The next best moment was the birth of Ceara, who was worth every minute of suffering I went through my entire life. I gave birth to a baby girl after only three hours of easy labor. It was the only thing about my life that's been easy. It's a miracle. A lot of people call it weight loss surgery. I look at it as life-giving surgery. Without the surgery, without Dr. Flancbaum, I wouldn't have my little girl. I give Dr. Flancbaum a lot of credit because he did the surgery well. I give me a lot of credit because I made the actual decision to go through with it. A lot of people say this surgery is taking the easy way out, but doing something drastic is never easy. My only regret is that I didn't have it sooner.

18

FREQUENTLY ASKED QUESTIONS

What is bariatric or weight loss surgery?

Bariatric surgery is the area of surgery that focuses on operations to reduce weight and treat obesity. The name comes from the Greek words *baros,* meaning weight, and *iatrike,* meaning treatment.

How is bariatric surgery different from liposuction?

Bariatric surgery is major surgery involving the gastrointestinal tract. The stomach and intestines are modified so that less food can be consumed or absorbed, which leads to a substantial loss of weight that can be maintained for years. Liposuction is a form of cosmetic surgery in which areas of the body are reshaped or re-sculpted by removing excess amounts of fat in those areas. The purpose of liposuction is not to produce weight loss.

How do I know if I'm a candidate for this surgery?

You must have clinically severe obesity, also known as morbid obesity. This means your BMI must be higher than 40, or you must be at least 100 lbs. above your ideal body weight. You may be a candidate if you're less than 100 pounds overweight, if you also have significant health problems due to your weight, such as type II diabetes. Most people with clinically severe obesity are good candidates for surgical treatment—as long as you understand the procedure, don't have a severe, pathological eating disorder, and are willing to come back for lifelong follow-up.

What is BMI?

It stands for Body Mass Index, and it determines someone's health risk related to their weight. A BMI greater than 40 or greater than 35 with associated medical problems means you have clinically severe obesity, which is associated with diabetes, heart disease, high blood pressure, high cholesterol, heartburn, gallstones, arthritis, urinary stress incontinence, infertility, and some types of cancer.

Does my weight alone justify such extreme measures?

Yes. Morbid obesity is an independent risk factor for premature death, with the risk rising as the BMI increases. People with a BMI of 30 have a relative risk of dying early that is 1.3 times greater than normal-weight individuals. By the time the BMI is 40, the risk is close to 3 times as great.

How do I calculate my BMI and Ideal Body Weight?

Ideal Body Weight is equal to 100 lbs. for the first 5 ft. + 5 lbs. for each additional inch for women, and 106 lbs. for the first 5 ft. + 6 lbs. for each additional inch for men. BMI can be calculated using the following formula: Multiply your weight in pounds by 705, then divide by the square of your height in inches. For example, if you weigh 130 pounds and are 5'4" (64 in.) tall, your BMI is $(130 \times 705) \div (64 \times 64) = 22.4$. (If you use the metric system, divide your weight in kilograms by the square of your height in meters.) There are also height and weight tables that tell you your BMI.

I feel so guilty about being obese . . . Is it all my fault?

No. Obesity tends to run in families. Identification of several genes and their corresponding hormones (leptin) has been found to be at least partially responsible for obesity. Therefore, there is evidence that obesity is at least partially biological, helping to change the misconception that it is a behavioral or psychological disorder. I consider obesity a disease that needs a cure, rather than a moral failing that is the fault of the individual.

Why should I consider WLS?

Because it works! Surgical treatment for obesity is the ONLY treatment that reliably produces significant and sustained weight loss. People with clinically severe obesity are at great risk for developing many associated medical conditions. Research has shown that surgical treatment results in significant weight loss and improvement in most problems associated with obesity. Surgical treatment for clinically severe obesity has been endorsed by the National Institutes of Health, the World Health Organization, Shape Up America!, the American Heart Association, the American Dietetic Association, and the American Obesity Association.

Why not just lose the weight through diet and exercise and skip the serious complications that could result from surgery?

If you can lose the necessary amount of weight (and keep it off) through diet and exercise—more power to you! Ninety-five percent of the people considering WLS have tried (sometimes numerous times) and failed. I like to use this analogy: If someone asks, "If I can buy a lottery ticket and win the lottery, why do I have to work for a living?" my answer would be, "You don't. If it is easier and less painful to win the lottery and you can do it, then go for it." For a morbidly obese individual, losing a significant amount of weight is comparable to winning the lottery.

Why not take drugs to combat obesity?

Drug treatment does produce limited success (usually weight loss of about 35 to 40 pounds). However, concerns about safety of long-term treatment have limited the drugs available and the length of time people can take them. This in turn limits their effectiveness because, as with any chronic disease, such as diabetes or high blood pressure, the drug is only effective as long as it is taken.

How does WLS promote weight loss?

Operations for the treatment of obesity usually induce weight loss by limiting the amount of food consumed, altering the normal absorption of nutrients, and/or altering the way the body utilizes energy. A Roux-en-Y gastric bypass does all three. It actually boosts your metabolism for the first eighteen months, which is one reason patients lose weight so quickly.

Is it unhealthy to lose weight rapidly after WLS?

I like to answer this question by asking another question: "Is it healthy to be 100 pounds overweight?" The rapid weight loss experienced after WLS is extremely gratifying psychologically and physically. If you eat properly, making sure you get enough protein, there should be no ill effects from it.

How do I find a doctor who performs WLS?

Ask your primary-care physician for a referral or contact the American Society for Bariatric Surgery (see Appendix A: Resources) and ask for a surgeon in your area. Go to the surgeon's support groups and talk to his patients to find out what their experiences have been. Ask for patients you can call for references. If there is a teaching hospital in your area, see if they have a bariatric-surgery program. If you have access to the Web, visit the Websites listed at the back of this book and you can find links to many bariatric surgical practices.

Selecting a physician is a difficult decision. What qualities should I look for in a surgeon?

Look for a person who is committed to caring for severely obese patients. Obesity is a chronic disease and it requires specialized pre-operative care and post-operative follow-up. The surgeon should not delegate these to other individuals.

What is a bariatric surgeon?

The field of obesity surgery is also known as bariatric surgery. Bariatric surgeons are general surgeons who perform surgical procedures in the abdominal cavity.

Do the surgeon's skills and experience make a difference in the outcome of the surgery?

Of course. The more experience a surgeon has with a particular operation, the better he or she usually performs it.

If I'm not happy with the results, can the operation be reversed?

Only in an emergency. Any weight loss procedure should be thought of as a permanent solution, because if it is reversed, the weight will be regained. Although technically feasible, reoperative surgery is much more difficult and complex and the result will NOT, in all likelihood, restore the individual to the exact same state as before surgery. This can be thought of as similar to remodeling a house. If you knock down walls and add rooms and floors, it's usually permanent. Although they can be knocked down again, such a procedure would typically be very involved and the result not necessarily identical to the original.

Can you explain exactly what you do, in terms that I can understand, when you perform a Roux-en-Y gastric bypass?

The Roux-en-Y gastric bypass (RYGB) is a combination of a restrictive (inhibiting the amount of food that can be eaten) and a malabsorptive (limiting the amount of food that is absorbed into the system) procedure. The restrictive component consists of creating a small pouch at the top of the stomach with a surgical stapler. The malabsorptive portion is created by dividing the small intestine and rerouting it so that one portion is connected to the small stomach pouch (Roux-limb) and the remaining portion, which delivers the bile and pancreatic juice, is reconnected to the small intestine at a predetermined distance from the stomach.

What is a VBG?

Vertical banded gastroplasty (VBG), which is only restrictive, is another common form of WLS. This operation is performed by creating a one-ounce pouch near the junction of the stomach and esophagus using a vertically placed staple line.

Which operation do you prefer and why?

I prefer the Roux-en-Y gastric bypass (RYGB) because it produces greater weight loss more reliably than the vertical banded gastroplasty (VBG), and the weight lost is more likely to stay off.

At last weigh-in, I was 450 pounds. Is there any limit on how heavy one can be to have obesity surgery?

No. I have successfully operated on a patient who weighed 750 lbs. and had a BMI of 100. The operative risks are higher the more you weigh, but they still don't approach the risk of remaining at such a high weight.

How much weight can one expect to lose after surgery?

Most patients lose between 50 and 70 percent of their excess body weight over about 1 to 1½ years. Some reach their ideal weight, but most don't.

Can you gain the weight back?

Long-term results after Roux-en-Y gastric bypass have shown that patients usually regain less than 15 percent of the weight they lost after ten years. However, if you go back to your old eating habits and don't exercise at all, you might gain more than that.

How long does it take to perform the operation?

The open Roux-en-Y gastric bypass usually takes between one and two hours, depending on the surgeon. The VBG should take less time and the BPD or DS (described in Chapter 7), which is more complex, should take longer.

Does it matter how long it takes? I'd be asleep anyway.

The length of the operation may make a difference. Many studies have documented an increase in the incidence of infectious complications, such as pneumonia and wound infection, after prolonged surgical procedures. Longer operations result in a fall in body temperature that interferes with the immune system. In addition, longer operative times mean increased exposure to general anesthesia, which often results in the collapse of portions of the lung and can lead to pneumonia. In general, shorter operations are safer.

How long will I be in the hospital? How long does it take to recuperate?

Most patients are admitted to the hospital on the morning of surgery, remain in the hospital for two or three days, and require between two and six weeks to recuperate before returning to work, depending upon the type of job they have.

Will I have to stay until I've had a bowel movement?

I don't require my patients to stay in the hospital until they have had a bowel movement, although some surgeons do. But constipation or diarrhea should be reported to your surgeon so they can be appropriately treated.

I'm concerned about my future. Does anyone know what adverse long-term effects Roux-en-Y surgery will have on me?

The only long-term adverse effects of Roux-en-Y surgery are vitamin and iron deficiencies. These can be treated with vitamins, iron, and B12 supplements.

When I tell people that I'm considering this operation, they all have something negative to say. Why does WLS seem to have such a bad reputation?

The operations that were performed thirty years ago achieved weight loss but carried a high complication and mortality rate. That's when the surgery acquired a bad reputation, and rightly so. We no longer perform those operations. The ones done currently achieve comparable weight loss and are safe.

I really like to eat. What's going to stop me from overeating after the surgery?

Because your stomach will be smaller, it will fill up with food sooner. When the food touches the walls of the stomach, it sends a message to the brain that you don't want any more to eat. The brain will receive this signal after eating much less food, and consequently you'll eat less. Most people just don't feel as hungry. When you do overeat, or eat too quickly, you may experience what's called "dumping syndrome."

What is dumping, and does everybody have it after WLS?

Dumping is a phenomenon that can occur after stomach surgery, in which the food is short-circuited into the small intestine, bypassing the normal route of passage through the pylorus, which regulates its release into the intestine. The rapid passage of simple sugars or fat molecules into the small intestine then causes the release of several chemicals and hormones that can produce nausea, vomiting, abdominal cramps, and diarrhea. Not everyone experiences dumping after a gastric bypass, and no one should after a VBG or DS. If you do, consult with your surgeon or nutritionist to modify your diet.

A year after the surgery, are most people generally happier with their lives?

Yes, much happier. Most patients say they would do it again "in a heartbeat." Studies show that this kind of patient satisfaction is a true test of the surgery.

When it's over, will there be things I need to do after surgery?

Regular long-term follow-up is needed to monitor weight loss, provide dietary counseling, and monitor for the occurrence of nutritional deficiencies or complications.

I'm sixteen years old. Can someone be too young to be a candidate for this surgery?

Yes. People can be too young. You need to have stopped growing and you must have a mature bone age. In addition, you must understand the surgery and want it. You can't have an operation because your friends or your parents want you to. You need to be able to give informed consent, which means you make an educated decision and then give your permission for the procedure. It is also necessary that your parents are supportive of your decision and understand the role they will need to play in your care and recovery.

I'm well over fifty. Can you be too old for this surgery?

Age is one factor that needs to be considered together with all other aspects of a person's health. I would not give an arbitrary or absolute cutoff. I have done gastric bypasses on several patients in their late sixties and early seventies, with excellent results.

I am severely overweight, have diabetes, hypertension, and congestive heart failure. My internist tells me that I am "too sick" to be a candidate for WLS.

If you are overweight with associated problems due to obesity, you are not too sick to have this operation! You are too sick NOT to have it. The only chance you have for improvement in your medical conditions is through weight loss.

What's the difference between an open RYGB and a laparoscopic RYGB? Which is best?

Until recently, all abdominal operations were performed through an incision that opened the abdomen, providing exposure to the internal structures. Laparoscopy is a method by which the surgical procedures can be performed through a series of small incisions using specifically made instruments guided by a video camera. Like all methods, laparoscopy has certain advantages and disadvantages that should be understood and considered. The advantage of laparoscopy in WLS is related to the size of the incision. The disadvantages of laparoscopy include a considerably longer operating time (which poses increased risk of certain serious complications), significant technical difficulties in performing the procedure that frequently lead to compromises in technique, and increased cost of equipment and personnel. At this point in time, based upon the scientific data available, I do not believe that one method is clearly better than the other. The one that is best in any given situation is the one that your surgeon is most comfortable performing safely.

Will I need vitamins after surgery? What kind should I take, and when?

After Roux-en-Y surgery, most surgeons recommend vitamins. Some routinely prescribe iron and vitamin B_{12} as well. I prescribe prenatal vitamins post-operatively and then follow the patients post-operatively for iron and vitamin B_{12} deficiencies, the most common deficiencies that they experience. You should also make sure to take supplemental calcium, since osteoporosis is a potential long-term complication.

Why are vitamins necessary? Can't I get all my nutrition from food, once I can eat a reasonable amount again?

Due to the bypass of most of the stomach and the upper part of the small intestine, some nutrients aren't absorbed properly from food. You have to take a substantial amount extra to have enough absorption.

Will I need monthly vitamin B12 injections?

Oral vitamin B_{12} is less efficient and reliable than injections. However, you can buy sublingual vitamin B_{12} that dissolves under the tongue, which is better than the pill form. There is also a new nasal spray called Nascobal that delivers vitamin B_{12} directly into the body, bypassing the stomach. It's available by prescription. If you become deficient, you must have injections, but these are easy and can even be done at home once a month.

Will I need a blood transfusion?

It is unusual for a patient to require a blood transfusion during WLS, but some patients have their own blood stored prior to surgery, just in case.

What pre-operative testing should be done?

I ask for routine lab studies, a chest X ray, and an electrocardiogram. If other tests are indicated (based on those results or on the physical exam and history), then those are performed as well.

I've heard about "sleep studies." What are they all about?

Obstructive sleep apnea and obesity hypoventilation syndrome are among the most dangerous complications of severe obesity. Patients with symptoms of these disorders, such as snoring, daytime sleepiness, and observed periods in which they stop breathing, should have a sleep study to rule out sleep apnea.

If I have sleep apnea, how will this affect me?

Twenty percent of patients who undergo WLS have mild to moderate sleep apnea. Their level of apnea should have no significant effect during or after the operation. However, patients with severe sleep apnea should have their oxygen-saturation level monitored during and after the surgery. Patients who normally use a nocturnal CPAP or BIPAP should use these treatments in the hospital (although some surgeons feel this is unnecessary).

Should my surgeon perform a physical examination? What will he/she be looking for?

Yes, your surgeon should perform an exam. He/she will be looking for any factors that might complicate surgery. If he/she knows what to expect beforehand, potential problems can be avoided.

Do I have to do anything special the day(s) before surgery?

All I require of my patients is that they not eat or drink after midnight the night before the surgery. However, some surgeons require longer periods without food or drink, or bowel preps such as those performed before a colonoscopy.

Will I have a tube up my nose after surgery? I find the prospect really frightening.

Some surgeons require what's called an NG tube even after you wake up, until they are sure there are no leaks. However, I do not require one, and many other surgeons don't either. If you do have one, don't be concerned. Patients tell me the NG tube is really no big deal until its removal, which is mildly uncomfortable.

What is a leak, and how do you prevent one?

A leak occurs when one of the suture or staple lines closing off the intestine or connecting two parts of the intestine does not hold. This allows digestive juices that are normally inside the intestine to "leak" into the abdominal cavity, where they can cause severe irritation and infection, similar to that which occurs with a perforated ulcer or a ruptured appendix. Leaks can occur after any intestinal surgery and are no more common following WLS. The only way to prevent leaks is by employing safe surgical techniques. Most surgeons check for leaks during surgery by injecting air or a colored solution into the stomach and seeing if anything leaks out. However, this is not foolproof and only checks for openings in the suture and staple lines in the stomach. Many surgeons also check for leaks post-operatively before initiating feedings with an upper-GI study, in which gastrograffin (a liquid that can be seen on an X ray) is swallowed and X-ray pictures are taken.

Should I have psychological testing? If so, should it be through the doctor's office or on my own?

Mental health is part of overall health. If a patient has a history of mental illness, then it would be irresponsible to operate on that patient without a consultation with a psychologist or psychiatrist, just as it would be irresponsible to operate on someone with a history of heart disease without a consultation with a cardiologist. It is necessary to rule out disorders like anorexia and bulimia, which are contraindications for surgery. In some cases, psychological testing is not clinically indicated. However, if your insurance company requires it, you'll have to comply. Have the testing done by a licensed psychologist or psychiatrist who is convenient for you.

I smoke. I would like to quit—but I haven't. How will smoking affect me?

In addition to the well-known ill effects of smoking, it can complicate surgery by increasing the incidence of pneumonia and pulmonary problems immediately after surgery. I recommend that patients stop smoking at least several weeks before surgery.

What's an epidural, and should I have one?

An epidural is a type of anesthetic administered by placing a needle and a catheter in the back adjacent to the spinal canal. It is similar to a spinal anesthetic or a spinal tap. Its purpose is to provide pain relief over the abdominal area (not as anesthesia during surgery). The choice of whether or not to have another (less invasive) form of post-operative pain relief, such as a patient-controlled morphine pump, is up to the patient and surgeon. In my practice I do not use epidurals.

I don't like pain. (Does anyone?) How much pain can I expect? What kind of pain will it be? What will alleviate it?

All operations are associated with pain. Typically the pain is worst the first day or two and then it gets better. In the hospital, my patients use a morphine pump, which is a device that allows them to control the amount of pain medication they receive. I send them home with oral pain medication, usually containing codeine.

Should the anesthesiologist be experienced with obese people?

That's just common sense. The more experience an anesthesiologist has intubating and managing obese patients, the better. For instance, there can be problems locating the airway of an obese patient that an experienced anesthesiologist will know how to overcome.

Will my gallbladder be removed at the same time?

Maybe yes. Maybe no. There is a strong relationship between obesity and gallstones and a high incidence of gallbladder attacks during rapid weight loss in patients with gallstones. For this reason, it is customary for patients to be screened for gallstones before surgery. Patients with documented gallstones should have their gallbladders removed at the time of surgery.

Will I be in the Intensive Care Unit (ICU) after surgery?

Some surgeons admit their patients to the ICU. I have found this practice unnecessary if all goes smoothly.

Will I need to be catheterized after surgery?

A urinary catheter is a plastic tube inserted into the bladder to drain all of the urine into a collection bag. This allows doctors to measure the exact amount of urine made, which provides information about how the heart and kidneys are functioning. In routine cases, such information can be obtained by using other measures. There is a risk of urinary-tract infection from using catheters, which can slow recovery and prolong hospitalization. Although some surgeons use them routinely, in my practice I rarely find them necessary. Plus, needing to use the bathroom will motivate a patient to get out of bed and move after surgery— which is important for recovery.

Will I have an IV? Where will it be placed?

Yes. All patients having major surgery require an IV to receive fluid and drugs. It can usually be placed in the arm, but sometimes in obese patients where veins cannot be located, it needs to be placed under the collarbone.

What is an A-line (besides a subway and a dress), and will I need one?

An arterial line (A-line) is similar to an IV and is usually placed in the wrist. It allows for constant measurement of blood pressure during the operation and allows the anesthesiologist to sample the blood oxygen levels. There is some risk involved, so most surgeons use it selectively in patients who have heart problems or severe sleep apnea.

I'm scared that I could get a blood clot. My mother once had one after an operation. What do you do to prevent them?

Typically, patients are given a blood-thinning drug such as heparin to reduce the risk of clots before and after surgery. An inflatable device is also often employed on the legs and thighs to increase circulation, thereby decreasing the risk of clots.

I've had some heart problems. How likely is it that I'll have a heart attack when I have this surgery?

Cardiac problems can occur after any major operation but are more common in patients who already have angina, heart failure, hypertension, high cholesterol, and diabetes. Myocardial infarction (heart attack) is extremely rare. A more common problem in this population is "sudden cardiac death," which is caused by a sudden change in the rhythm of the heart. Severely obese patients are at about an eight times greater risk for this complication than normal-weight individuals. This may not be a preventable complication, although some individuals have findings on their electrocardiogram (ECG) that can be a warning sign.

Why do some people get pneumonia after surgery?

Patients undergoing abdominal operations under general anesthesia sometimes experience a collapse of a small portion of their lungs. This collapse is termed *atelectasis* and typically manifests itself as a fever on the night of surgery. This usually resolves with simple maneuvers such as early ambulation (walking), coughing, and deep-breathing exercises and chest physiotherapy. Untreated atelectasis can progress to pneumonia if the collapsed portions are not reexpanded. Pneumonia is a more serious complication, requiring antibiotic treatments and a prolonged hospitalization. The incidence of pneumonia is low if the operation is completed in under ninety minutes and appropriate precautions are aggressively instituted.

Can I develop ulcers as a result of WLS?

Sometimes. In the RYGB and other operations, a portion of the small intestine is sewn to the stomach. This connection is not normal, and the small intestine is therefore prone to develop ulcers called marginal ulcers from the strong acid contained in the stomach. Most of these ulcers can be treated successfully with medication. It is helpful if post-op patients avoid drugs that irritate the stomach, such as aspirin, ibuprofen, and naproxen sodium.

My mother's cousin had WLS and then developed a wound infection. Can that be a complication?

Obese patients have thick abdominal walls and are prone to wound infections. The incidence can be as high as 10 percent, compared to a 2 percent rate in normal-weight patients. Wound infections are not life-threatening, but their treatment is time-consuming and can delay recovery. Precautions can be taken to prevent many wound infections. All patients undergoing

WLS should receive prophylactic (preventive) antibiotics, which are administered before surgery and continued for the day of the operation. In my practice, I have been able to reduce the rate of wound infections to about 2 percent by leaving a drain in the subcutaneous fat to suck out the fluid that accumulates. In addition, I close the skin with a continuous plastic-surgery stitch, which does not require removal and is more cosmetically appealing.

I've heard that incisional hernia is a common complication of WLS. What causes this?

An incisional hernia is caused by a defect in the abdominal wall through which fat or intestine can protrude. Incisional hernias occur in up to 15 percent of patients after obesity surgery. A huge amount of tension is placed upon the stitches holding the abdomen closed in severely obese patients, and either the tissue or stitches do not hold. Most incisional hernias will slowly continue to enlarge over time and will ultimately need surgery to repair. The good news is that insurance will often pay for a tummy tuck as part of the hernia repair.

Can I die as a result of WLS?

It's possible, but unlikely. The risk of death in large groups of patients undergoing WLS is about 1 percent, or one out of a hundred patients. Although the risk may vary from patient to patient depending upon each individual's overall health, it is impossible to predict which patients will die. However, clinically severe obesity is a life-threatening condition and many patients have associated medical problems, such as sleep apnea, hypertension, coronary artery disease, and diabetes, that increase this risk. In my opinion, the patients who are the sickest as a result of their obesity need this surgery the most. They are risking death just being morbidly obese, since there are no other effective treatments to offer them.

We've talked a lot about potential negative side effects. Is there anything positive I can expect soon after surgery?

Glad you asked that. Weight loss by any means often results in considerable improvement or complete resolution of most obesity-related medical conditions. The degree of improvement is not necessarily related to the amount of weight loss. "Improvement" refers to a reduced requirement for treatment, whereas "complete resolution" implies a cure. The effect of Roux-en-Y on type II diabetes is noteworthy. Dramatic improvement occurs in abnormalities associated with diabetes. Within days of surgery, fasting blood-sugar levels are normal, blood levels of insulin are lower, and most patients are able to be discharged without insulin. There is also improvement in hypertension, blood lipids, and sleep apnea in a large percentage of patients.

How long after surgery will I be allowed to drink liquids?

I allow my patients to drink liquids the first day after surgery, once I have ascertained that there has not been a leak.

What is a stomach binder, and should I wear one after surgery? Will it help with the pain?

A stomach binder is a device similar to a girdle. It makes some patients more comfortable. If it helps you, by all means wear it.

What will I be able to eat after surgery?

After the Roux-en-Y gastric bypass, most surgeons recommend liquids and blenderized or soft foods for the first four weeks or so after surgery. Emphasis should be on consuming foods high in protein, such as dairy products, and maintaining good hydration by drinking two to three quarts of liquid per day.

After surgery, will the doctor send me home with any medications?

Most patients leave the hospital with a variety of prescriptions. Pain medication, usually a codeine derivative, is routine. Often, these stronger pills can be alternated with acetaminophen if pain is not severe. Vitamins are frequently recommended. Individuals with intact gallbladders should be given Actigall in order to prevent the formation of gallstones caused by weight loss. Some surgeons also prescribe H_2-blockers, which reduce stomach acid and are helpful in preventing marginal-ulcer formation.

Would you recommend telling my employer that I am having WLS? Should I try to keep this a secret?

This is a personal decision. If you feel that the fact that you are having WLS will negatively affect you in the workplace, you are free to keep it quiet. However, the more people who understand that obesity is a disease that can be treated surgically, the better for the status of the obese segment of the population.

How do I select a hospital in my area?

If possible, try to select a hospital that has a commitment to the treatment of obesity. There are a few questions you can ask to determine if that level of commitment is present. Does the hospital have special equipment designed to accommodate obese individuals, such as hospital gowns that fit properly and bathrooms and chairs that are large enough? Does the hospital have a team of professionals to offer appropriate post-operative follow-up care? Are the nurses on the floor trained to take care of obese patients? If the answers to these questions are yes, then you've found the right hospital.

There is no surgeon near me that does this surgery. Should I travel to have it?

It is always preferable to have the surgery near home, but if you have no other choice, yes. Just make sure your primary-care physician and your surgeon are willing to communicate about your care post-op.

While I'm in the hospital can I use the over-the-counter medications that I regularly use?

Discuss any over-the-counter medications with your surgeon. He or she will decide if they are appropriate for you to take. In general, it is best to avoid aspirin or aspirinlike anti-inflammatory drugs such as ibuprofen or naproxen sodium (known as NSAIDs), because they can cause stomach ulcers.

I snore and I don't want to keep a roommate awake. Will I have a private room?

Most likely not. It depends on what your insurance will cover and what the hospital has available.

Can a friend or family member stay with me while I'm in the hospital?

Not usually, but it depends on the hospital. Some hospitals these days are making arrangements for family members to stay with patients after surgery. Hopefully, you will be in a hospital that has nursing staff experienced with taking care of patients who have had WLS.

How long after surgery will I be able to walk around?

The nurses will get you up and around as soon as possible, possibly right after you get back to your room from the recovery room. This will reduce the chances of you accumulating fluid in your lungs, contracting pneumonia, and developing blood clots.

I have bracelets and rings that won't come off. Will I need to have these cut off? How about dentures?

I'm afraid so. Jewelry and removable dentures cannot be worn into the operating room.

Have you ever heard of a case where surgery couldn't be performed after it was started because of some unforeseen complication?

Very rarely, a surgeon may encounter an anatomical problem that would preclude completing the operation or, more likely, identify another medical problem, such as a tumor, that would be more important and cause him or her to abandon the weight loss procedure.

Will my hair fall out? If so, when will it start falling out? How much? When will it grow back?

Hair loss after WLS is fairly common if the weight loss is extremely rapid. People who lose weight more slowly tend not to lose hair. The hair will grow back when the rapid weight loss period is over—usually about six to nine months after surgery. However, unlike chemotherapy, WLS does not cause baldness, just thinning. Although protein deficiency is probably the most common cause of hair loss, iron deficiency can contribute as well. Increasing protein and iron intake will improve the situation, although it may take several months to resolve.

I have heard that there is a lot of diarrhea and stinky gas after the surgery. How can I minimize it?

Diarrhea and excess gas (flatulence) are rare (less than 5 percent of patients) and usually occur only after more-distal gastric bypasses or the bilio-pancreatic diversion (BPD) and duodenal switch (DS). They are usually related to malabsorption of fat, but can rarely be the result of bacterial overgrowth within the intestine (blind loop). In the case of a blind loop, antibiotics may be helpful.

Will I vomit a lot?

Vomiting is more common after gastroplasty (VBG) than after gastric bypass. Some vomiting (or retching) during the first few weeks after surgery may be expected, but persistent vomiting should be evaluated to rule out an ulcer, stricture, or obstruction.

I really like to eat out with my friends. Will I be able to go to restaurants after this surgery?

Yes, after a few months when your diet has normalized, you should be able to enjoy eating in restaurants—but you'll be eating smaller portions.

How soon after surgery will I be able to lift heavy objects? When will I be able to drive?

The danger of lifting after surgery has to do with the risk of developing an incisional hernia. It takes incisions six weeks to fully heal, so the longer one waits, the better. Mild lifting can be done fairly soon, but it is probably preferable to wait the full amount of time before lifting heavier objects. Although the incisions following laparoscopy are smaller than after open surgery, the same risks do apply. I allow patients to drive after surgery when they are pain free and no longer require narcotics. This decision relates to their ability to control the vehicle and road safety, not healing from surgery.

Another embarrassing question: After surgery, when can I resume my sex life?

It is probably safe to resume sexual activity when one is pain free.

My husband is worried that when I become smaller, other men will suddenly be interested in me. How will losing all of this weight affect my relationships?

Relationships can change after any life-altering event. Many obese people attract friends and mates who want a nonthreatening partner. Once you become slim and good-looking, people in your life may feel competitive and threatened by your transformation. In some cases, it may be appropriate to seek counseling to help you adjust to your new body and to changes in your relationships.

When can I bathe or shower?

I allow patients to shower after 48 hours, when the incision has "sealed" so that water cannot seep in.

Will I need help performing any activities of daily living such as using the bathroom or dressing?

Patients may need some assistance with these activities in the early post-operative period but can usually manage fairly well after a few days. There is much individual variation among people, and it is really difficult to generalize.

What is helpful to have on hand after surgery?

Many patients recommend a long wooden spoon to wrap toilet paper around so they can wipe themselves after a bowel movement, since the incision makes this task difficult. Most patients find it humiliating to have to ask a nurse or family member to do this for them. Also, some patients like to have a recliner at home to sleep in for a while, because getting out of a flat bed can be painful at first. Bring loose clothes to the hospital, so you will have something comfortable to wear on the way home.

I know that the staples you use to close the incision inside are there permanently. How long will the outside staples stay in?

This is highly variable among surgeons. Most surgeons will leave skin staples in until the first post-op office visit, which may be between one and two weeks after discharge. I currently do not use skin staples at all. I use a subcuticular closure with absorbable (dissolving) sutures, which is more cosmetically appealing and does not require suture removal.

How long do I need someone to stay with me after the surgery?

I would advise having someone to be with you for several days after you are discharged from the hospital. You shouldn't need a great deal of care—but it's good to have someone around in case of any kind of complication.

I know that I'm never going to wear a bikini. But what will my scar look like?

With open surgery, the scar usually begins at the bottom of the breastbone and may extend as low as the belly button. With laparoscopy, there are usually five or six small incisions, measuring ¼ to 1½ inches in length, which eventually disappear, leaving little or no scarring.

How small will my stomach pouch be, and will it stretch back out?

This depends upon how small your surgeon makes it, which varies from surgeon to surgeon and with each operation. In general, surgeons who perform VBG and gastric bypasses make pouches that hold about one ounce. The stomach after a biliopancreatic diversion or duodenal switch holds four to six ounces, because these operations work differently. The pouch will stretch out somewhat over time but should stay small enough to substantially restrict what you eat.

I really love eating sweets. How will eating sugar affect me?

Sugars will only affect you if you have a gastric bypass, in which case you may experience dumping. However, most patients after gastric bypass lose their taste for sweets. There are some that do retain their sweet tooth. These patients have to carefully watch their intake of sweets or risk regaining weight. The ability to eat unlimited amounts of sweets after a VBG is one of the reasons this surgery is less effective than an RYGB.

Will dairy products upset my stomach?

Only if you have lactose intolerance. Diabetics need to be aware of the sugar content in milk.

I'm a big popcorn fan. Will there be foods that I can never eat?

Actually, patients say that popcorn is the one food that goes down really easily. After a VBG, there are many foods that people cannot eat because they cause vomiting. Some of these include meat, pasta, certain fruits and vegetables that have "skin," or foods with larger-size bites. After gastric bypass, most patients develop an aversion to extremely sweet and high-fat foods (which can cause dumping if eaten), and some may have trouble with meat early on, but this usually resolves over time. However, results are individual and one patient may have trouble with pizza while another can't tolerate beans. Some can eat everything. It's very hard to predict.

Would you recommend that I join a support group?

Support groups can be helpful. People sometimes need to discuss their feelings with others who are "in the same boat." Support groups that are facilitated by mental-health professionals and individuals with expertise about the procedure, such as the surgeon or dietitian, are ideal. It is important attendees not come away with misinformation and unrealistic expectations.

How do you feel about Internet support groups?

Internet support groups can be helpful in obtaining practical hints. They're a great place to form relationships with people who are dealing with the same issues. On the other hand, there is a great deal of misinformation on the Internet. I guess a good rule would be, just because you see it online doesn't make it accurate.

Should I take protein supplements?

Most patients do not require protein supplements. After a restrictive operation, since you eat less, what you eat is important. Therefore, you should pay attention to eating healthfully, emphasizing foods with high protein content. However, if you find yourself snacking on junk food, you would be better off having a protein shake or bar. Look for products with low sugar and fat content.

How often should I weigh myself? Will I be subject to plateaus?

As often as you like, but I would caution about becoming obsessed with your weight loss and the rate of weight loss. It may be variable, and plateaus can occur. This is a long process, often lasting between 1½ and 2 years.

What kind of exercise should I do after surgery, and when can I begin?

It is good to begin exercising as early as you can post-operatively. Pace yourself and don't overdo it, especially if you have not been exercising regularly before surgery. Start with light aerobic exercise like walking, water aerobics, or an exercise bike and gradually increase to more-strenuous activities. Try to find an activity you enjoy so you'll stick with it.

Should I take the same dosages of prescription medications after my surgery since my absorption rate is changed?

In general, no changes in drug dosage are required. Some medications, such as thyroid medication, may require adjustment. Of course, any medications you are taking for diabetes will have to be reduced or eliminated.

Sometimes my joints ache. Will I ever be able to take anti-inflammatory drugs again? If not, what can I take instead?

I prefer that my patients avoid anti-inflammatory drugs permanently because of the risk of stomach irritation and ulcers. This is usually possible because the weight loss produces tremendous relief of the pressure on the joints and bones. Usually, acetaminophen will suffice. If anti-inflammatory drugs are needed, there are new prescription drugs called Celebrex and Vioxx that have the anti-inflammatory properties of aspirin and ibuprofen and may not irritate the stomach as much. If you must take an anti-inflammatory, you should take a proton pump inhibitor like Prilosec, Protonix, or Prevacid to help prevent stomach irritation. Some patients can have improvement from taking chondroitin and glucosamine to help rebuild damaged or destroyed cartilage.

I'm anxious to start a family after I lose some weight. Will this surgery affect my ability to become pregnant or carry a baby to term?

In fact, fertility problems improve with weight loss. Carrying a baby to term is safe after WLS; however, it is recommended that women use birth control and avoid becoming pregnant while they are still losing weight.

After the surgery should I wear a medic-alert bracelet?

I do not think this is necessary.

Money is tight. What will be the total cost of the surgery?

Hopefully, your insurance company will pick up most of the cost of the surgery. If you don't have private insurance, Medicaid may pay. When you think of your own outlay of money, all that you've spent on diets that haven't worked, if you have to pay for part of the surgery, it will surely be cost-effective. In addition, the health complications linked to obesity could keep you from working in the future, which would put you in a worse financial situation. The precise cost of the surgery and hospitalization varies throughout the country.

I'm so frustrated with my insurance company. Why do they make it so difficult to get approval?

Probably because they are not as educated as they should be. In the long run, not paying for WLS will cost them more money as obese patients inevitably become sicker.

I'm not too assertive and I don't have lots of spare time. What is the best and fastest way to try to get approval for the surgery?

Your surgeon simply needs to send a letter documenting the medical necessity of surgery to your insurance company. Beyond that, some carriers have specific requirements that will need to be addressed, such as a psychological evaluation, prescribed period of documented medically supervised weight loss attempts, etc.

Who can help during the appeal phase if my insurance refuses the first request?

Your surgeon should write another letter specifically addressing the reasons for the denial.

If my insurance will pay a percentage of the cost and I will have to assume a percentage, will the surgeon and the hospital accept payments? I can't possibly afford to pay a lump sum.

Payment arrangements and options will vary from doctor to doctor and hospital to hospital. However, you will find someone to work with you if you keep looking. Many bariatric surgeons understand how difficult it is to get covered and do want to help patients.

I've never been successful with a diet in the past. I've always gained back every pound I've lost. How do I know this surgery will work for me? How do I know I won't sabotage it just like I've sabotaged every other diet I've been on?

You don't. But it is a powerful physical tool to help you restrain your compulsive overeating. It actually changes the taste buds of many post-ops, and they lose their desire for sweets and fatty foods. There is a strong behavior-modification component, where overeating will cause you to feel ill or vomit. The tiny stomach you have will not allow you to eat huge quantities. You will certainly not be able to eat the quantities at one time that you used to eat. However, many people do sabotage this surgery by constant grazing. It is possible to gain weight back.

Will I get to my ideal weight with WLS?

Less than 5 percent of patients reach their ideal weight. Most lose 50 to 75 percent of their excess weight and keep it off five years or more. This statistic, though disappointing to many, is much better than the 95 percent who regain almost all of their lost weight and then some after dieting.

What about butter? Will I be able to have butter or will the fat in it cause dumping? And they say to eat eggs and cheese for protein, but eggs and cheese are fattening, right?

Everyone's tolerance for sweet and fatty foods is different. You'll probably be able to have butter in small quantities. Eggs do not generally cause dumping and are a good source of low-calorie protein. If you like cheese, you're better off with the fat-free or low-fat brands.

Will I be able to have fountain drinks? Carbonated drinks supposedly stretch your pouch. Is this true?

You're better off without soda, but it's really not clear if carbonated beverages cause the pouch to stretch. If you do drink soda, make it diet, and don't drink it with meals.

Will I still be hungry after surgery?

This is extremely individual. Many patients report an extreme reduction in hunger; others are hungry all the time. Sometimes the hunger abates after a year or so. If you're in the "hungry" category, you need to manage your food intake so that you eat smaller amounts more frequently.

How much intestine should be bypassed with a gastric bypass? What is a distal versus a proximal? Which is better?

Surgeons generally bypass two to five feet of intestine with an RYGB. Some surgeons vary the length of the bypass based on the BMI of the patient, usually bypassing more intestine in those heavier patients with BMIs greater than 50. Shorter bypasses are called proximal; longer are called distal. It appears that for people with BMIs less than 50, the length of the bypass doesn't matter. However, in people with BMIs greater than 50, longer bypasses may be better. More research needs to be done in this area.

RESOURCES

ORGANIZATIONS

American Society for Bariatric Surgery
www.asbs.org

7328 W. University Drive, Suite F
Gainesville FL 32607
(352) 331-4900 (phone)
(352) 331-4975 (fax)
E-mail: info@asbs.org

A comprehensive site to learn about the pros and cons of bariatric surgery. The ASBS is the premier professional organization of bariatric surgeons and allied health professionals with a strong interest in bariatric surgery.

Features:
- "Rationale for the Surgical Treatment of Morbid Obesity," a paper covering many aspects of surgery
- Membership listing of bariatric surgeons by state and city. Many listings are directly linked to physician Websites
- An interactive BMI calculator
- Links to other helpful sites

The International Federation for the Surgery of Obesity (IFSO)
www.obesity-online.com/ifso

An Internet location for an international society of bariatric surgeons. The IFSO is an international organization similar to the ASBS.

Features:
- Listing of professional meetings related to bariatric surgery
- "Statement on Morbid Obesity and its Treatment," a good introduction to the rationale for the surgical treatment of obesity
- "Patient Selection for Bariatric Surgery," a paper that helps prospective patients and their physicians determine who is a candidate for WLS

The American Obesity Association
1250 24th Street NW
Suite 300
Washington DC 20037
1-800-98-OBESE (1-800-986-2373)
or 202-776-7711
www.obesity.org

The AOA's mission is to educate the public about obesity, help health professionals to care for people with obesity, advocate for insurance coverage for obesity, fight for more funding for obesity research, end discrimination, and more. Membership in the AOA is open to the public.

Features include articles and information on:
- Obesity treatment
- Obesity and social security
- Hot issues, such as obesity and insurance, taxes, and medical deductions
- Other helpful materials

The American College of Surgeons
633 N Saint Clair Street
Chicago IL 60611-3211
(312) 202-5000 (telephone)
(312) 202-5001 (fax)
www.facs.org

The American College of Surgeons is a scientific and educational association of surgeons that was founded in 1913 to improve the quality of care for the surgical patient by setting high standards for surgical education and practice.

Members of the American College of Surgeons are referred to as "Fellows." The letters FACS (Fellow, American College of Surgeons) after a surgeon's name mean that the surgeon's education and training, professional qualifications, surgical competence, and ethical conduct have passed a rigorous evaluation and have been found to be consistent with the high standards established by the College.

Feature:
A search engine to find out if your surgeon is a member.

MAGAZINES AND JOURNALS (PRINT AND WEB)

Obesity Online
www.obesity-online.com

Obesity-Online is a multidisciplinary forum for research and treatment of massive obesity, including plastic surgery, psychiatry, endocrinology, nutrition, nursing, dietetics, and allied health fields.

Features:
Articles on physiology, internal medicine, psychology, surgery, fat discrimination
- Books
- Education
- Training centers
- Patient information

Obesity Surgery Including Laparoscopy and Allied Care is the official journal of the IFSO and the ASBS
www.obesitysurgery.com

Primarily of interest to surgeons and medical professionals, this journal features the latest research on every aspect of obesity surgery. It is not available on the Website but can be ordered there. Look up articles of interest in the library. The price makes it prohibitive to order.

Obesity Meds and Research News
www.obesity-news.com

An on-line magazine (subscription required) that provides comprehensive information on the latest medical therapies for obesity.

Features:
- Physician (mostly non-surgeon) finder listings
- Latest news about the treatment of obesity
- Latest news on pharmacotherapy and research into obesity's causes and cures

Obesity: Preventing and Managing the Global Epidemic Report of a World Health Organization Consultation
www.who.int/dsa/justpub/justpub.htm#Obesity

Technical Report Series, 2000, xii + 252 pages (English)
ISBN 92 4 120894 5
Sw.fr. 56.-/US $50.40
Order no. 1100894

This report records the conclusions and recommendations of a major WHO consultation convened to consider the alarming global epidemic of obesity, assess the magnitude of associated public-health problems, and map out strategies for prevention and control, including weight loss surgery. It includes a quote that supports weight loss surgery as the most effective weight reduction method for the severely obese.

BOOKS

Surgery for the Morbidly Obese Patient (out-of-print)
Mervyn Deitel
$39.50 (includes shipping and handling)
Send money order to:
FD-Communications
P.O. Box 62043
Victoria Terrace P.O.
North York ON M4A 2W1
Canada
Written in 1989. 400 pages. 32 chapters. 100 illustrations.

Fat No More
Norman B. Ackerman
Prometheus Books
Paperback $18.95

"Ackerman (emeritus, surgery, New York Medical College) examines the physical and psychological aspects of morbid obesity (over 100 pounds above ideal weight); discusses his personal experiences in treating such individuals; and offers some success stories. Based on 20 years of experience in the field, his writing is informed and informative and will be of interest to both a lay audience and the medical community." (review from booknews.com)

The Seven Secrets of Slim People
Vikki Hansen, M.S.W., and Shawn Goodman
HarperCollins
Paperback $5.99

Outlines a sensible program of dealing with emotional eating by paying attention to your body's hunger and satiety signals rather than dieting. Required reading for 007Secrets@egroups.com, a listserve of post-surgical patients dealing with eating problems in a nondiet context.

Going Under: Preparing Yourself for Anesthesia: Your Guide to Pain Control and Healing Techniques—Before, During and After Surgery
Monica W. Furlong and Elliot Essman
Autonomy Pub. Co.
Paperback $12.95

Gives brief histories and easy-to-read descriptions of local, general, and spinal anesthetics. Offers information on alternative systems of medicine, pain as a learned phenomena, anesthesia in childbirth, and healing, plus much more. It also offers a look at the medical field's bias against narcotics that forces some patients to "tough it out" instead of finding appropriate relief. Teaches about managing your postsurgical pain and helps you set realistic goals for your recovery.

Prepare for Surgery, Heal Faster
Peggy Huddleston and Christiane Northrup, M.D.
Angel River Press
Paperback $14.95
Audiocassette $8.95

This book and the accompanying cassette are highly recommended by readers who have been through surgery, including weight-loss-surgery patients. It has guided imagery and other meditation-type exercises that reduce anxiety pre-op and lessen pain and improve healing time post-op.

INSURANCE ASSISTANCE

Obesity Law and Advocacy Center
Walter Lindstrom
7710 Hazard Center Drive, Suite E, PMB No. 443
San Diego CA 92108
(619) 656-5251
www.obesitylaw.com

Tony C. Merry, Esq.
Palmer Volkema Thomas
140 E Town Street, Suite 1100
Columbus OH 43215
(614) 221-4400
Tmerry@pvtlaw.com

Mr. Merry is an expert in this area. He is willing to advise out-of-state clients and also takes cases on a contingency basis.

State Insurance Commissions on the Web
www.members.tripod.com/proagency/insurance3.html

Features:
A state-by-state listing of insurance departments and commissioners.

NUTRITIONAL INFORMATION

www.dietwatch.com

A helpful site with a nutrition calculator that helps you keep track of how much protein, fat, carbs, etc., you're eating.

POSITION PAPER WEBSITES
Use these statements to support your insurance claim.

NIH
Gastrointestinal Surgery for Severe Obesity. NIH Consensus Statement 1991 Mar 25–27;9(1):1–20.
http://text.nlm.nih.gov/nih/cdc/www/84txt.html

Text of the original NIH statement recommending WLS for morbid obesity.

American Obesity Association
http://www.shapeup.org/publications/guide2/app2.pdf

Concise description of the benefits and risks of WLS, including who is eligible, nutritional considerations, short-term and long-term outcomes.

American Dietetic Association
http://www.eatright.org/adap0197.html

Recommends WLS for patients with BMI over 40, or over 35 with co-morbid conditions.

American Heart Association
http://www.americanheart.org/Scientific/statements/1997/119701.html

Recommends WLS as "treatment of choice" when BMI is over 40.

MORE HELPFUL WEBSITES

Association for Morbid Obesity Support
http://www.obesityhelp.com/morbidobesity

One of the most comprehensive WLS sites on the Internet.

Features:
- A state-by-state physicians listing with patient recommendations
- Definition of terms used in bariatric surgery
- Comprehensive WLS library
- Faces of weight loss surgery—patients' stories
- Insurance information
- Postings of meetings and seminars
- Much more . . .

The Yahoogroups Obesity Surgery Support Groups (OSSG)
www.yahoogroups.com/community/OSSG

Plug OSSG into the search engine at yahoogroups.com and you will come up with a long list of listserves that deal with WLS. Their stated purpose is to discuss and offer support for physical and emotional issues as they relate to WLS for the morbidly obese. Topics covered include types of operations available, dietary guidelines, post-op reports, emotional, family, work, and recovery issues.

Offshoot groups include regional OSSG groups and groups organized by type of surgery, specific problems, pre-op and post-op concerns, and many other topics. Joining one or more of these lists is a good way to learn about WLS from people who've been there. Be wary, however, of possible misinformation. Most members of these groups have no medical background and may give advice based solely on their personal experience.

Duodenal-Switch Information Zone
http://www.duodenalswitch.com

A patient-hosted site for those who are interested in the duodenal-switch procedure. Provides information about the procedure, names of surgeons, FAQs, chat, links, patients' stories.

Carnie Wilson's On-Line Obesity Support Group
http://www.spotlighthealth.com/morbid_obesity/mo/mo.htm

Carnie Wilson's site, with the story of her successful weight loss surgery. Offers a support group, forum, chat, links, information on obesity.

About Obesity: The Physiology of Morbid Obesity
http://bandsters.crosswinds.net/About%20Obesity.htm

Collection of fascinating scientific and popular articles about morbid obesity with good links to other sites.

Olwen's Links
http://homepages.ihug.co.nz/~olwen

The home page of Olwen Williams, original moderator of the first OSSG list. Provides a lot of good information and links to many WLS programs.

Healthology.com
http://www.Healthology.com

Internet site dealing with many health issues. Contains videos and articles on WLS, including an interview with Dr. Flancbaum.

MITCH'S GOURMET RECIPES

Mitch Sewall writes a weekly cooking column for the *Woodstock Journal* in Woodstock, New York. He is an accomplished gourmet cook who has had a different kind of bypass—coronary bypass surgery. As a result he is experienced with low-fat cooking. He was kind enough to compile these wonderful high-protein, low-fat recipes for gastric bypass patients.

For information about his forthcoming book of recipes for WLS patients, e-mail him at Mitch-woodstock@aol.com.

Note: The serving sizes are based on 4-ounce portions of meat and 1-cup portions of vegetables and soups. Many WLS patients will not be able to eat this much, at least initially, but portion sizes take into consideration the need to feed a family of normal eaters. If you can only eat part of a portion, adjust the nutrient values accordingly.

SMOOTHIES

This is a master recipe for a high-protein smoothie. I have tried making them with all types of fruit. These are the best-tasting and easiest to make. Add whichever fruits you like. Egg whites appear in this master recipe because they are the best protein available—the standard to which other proteins are compared. Partially frozen milk and fruit make a thicker, richer smoothie.

Note: To destroy any harmful bacteria and/or salmonella, "coddle" the eggs. First boil eggs for 1 to 2 minutes and cool immediately to stop the cooking (otherwise you'll end up with a soft-boiled egg). If you get eggs from a reliable source it really isn't necessary to coddle them.

Master Recipe

2 egg whites (coddled or raw)
½–1 c. skim milk, partially frozen
1 tbsp. dry powdered fat-free milk (more protein)
2–3 tsp. artificial sweetener (or more to taste)
2 ice cubes

1. Into a blender, place egg whites, fruit, and ice cubes.
2. Begin blending at slow speed until fruit is pureed.
3. Slowly add the milk, powdered milk, and sweetener to the blender.
4. Now blend at high speed for at least 30 seconds.

Servings: 1

181 CAL. • 17 G PROTEIN • 27 G CARBOHYDRATE • ½ G FAT • 5 MG CHOLESTEROL

Cranberry Smoothie

Use about 1 cup almost completely frozen cranberry juice. (Pure cranberry juice is difficult to get these days; what one finds on the grocer's shelves is usually cranberry juice "cocktail," a mix of juice, water, and sugar.) If you can get the real thing, dilute it a bit and add 2 additional teaspoons of Equal or Splenda.

½ cup frozen skim milk

1. Add the juice slowly to the egg whites with the blender running at low speed.
2. Add remaining ingredients and continue as in master recipe.

Servings: 1

319 CAL. (THE CRANBERRY JUICE REALLY UPS THE CALORIE CONTENT) • 17 G PROTEIN •
62 G CARBOHYDRATE • ½ G FAT • 5 MG CHOLESTEROL

Strawberry Smoothie

1 pint of hulled and washed strawberries less ½ cup (or use the whole pint if you choose to). You may also use the frozen sweetened berries found in supermarkets, but omit the sweetener.

1. Partially freeze the berries. If using the frozen supermarket berries, partially thaw them.
2. Add remaining ingredients and follow master recipe.

260 CAL. • 18 G PROTEIN • 47 G CARBOHYDRATE • LESS THAN 1 G FAT •
5 MG CHOLESTEROL

Peach Smoothie

To master recipe add 2 large, very-ripe, skinned and pitted peaches. If fresh peaches are not in season, use 3 or more canned peach halves.

Note: To skin peaches, place peaches in boiling water for about 15 seconds. Remove with slotted spoon and immerse in cold water immediately or run under cold water. When cool, cut into the skin slightly and slip the skin right off the peaches.

1 serving

316 CAL. • 19 G PROTEIN • 62 G CARBOHYDRATE • 1 G FAT • 5 MG CHOLESTEROL

Note: A bit high in calories for a snack. This is okay if used as a meal.
Other fruits you can use: fresh or canned apricots; pitted, peeled, and sliced very ripe mango (I find this one fantastic); skinned and cored fresh pears or the canned variety. Try skinned and pitted papaya. Almost any washed berry can be used (if seeds bother you, stay away from raspberries or strain them once pureed).

Banana Eggnog

For a healthy high-protein snack, this "eggnog" hits the spot. To increase the protein content even more, you can add a tablespoon or two of powdered milk.

 1 c. nonfat or low-fat milk
 2 egg whites from coddled eggs (see note, above)
 1 peeled banana
 pinch of cinnamon and pinch of freshly grated nutmeg
 2 ice cubes

Place all in a blender. Blend at low speed, then increase speed to high for about 30 seconds. Pour into a glass and enjoy.

227 CAL. • 17 G PROTEIN • 7 G CARBOHYDRATE • 1 G FAT • 4.4 MG CHOLESTEROL

SOUPS, PUREES, AND SOFT FOODS

Aside from being easy to eat after surgery, soup always conjures feelings of satisfaction and hominess. It is the original comfort food. It is very easy to prepare and quite forgiving. Almost all of these soups contain beans as the major ingredient; hence they are high in protein. Many people don't realize just how much protein is found in beans. In years past beans were listed along with meats in any tables or books about nutrition. With so much protein they just didn't fit in with vegetables.

Old-Fashioned Pea Soup

A while ago I came across smoked neck bones in the meat department of my supermarket. I immediately thought of pea soup and how good these neck bones taste when cooked long and slowly. The smoky flavor also gets into the soup and enhances it. Almost any cut of smoked or salt-cured meat can be used. Traditionally it has always been a ham bone. Often I'll find smoked ham butts in the market at inexpensive prices; all of these marry well with pea soup. The best part is the mellow, moist, and tender meat that falls off the bone, which happens to be perfect for our diet. Also note that most soups and stews taste better after a day or two, so make enough to last a few days.

9 c. water (for a richer taste you can substitute chicken or
meat stock for some of the water)
2 c. green split peas
1 medium onion with root end cut off
1 garlic clove
1 stalk celery along with some leaves
2 tsp. salt
1 bay leaf
a ham bone or any of the other meat bones discussed above

1. Bring the water to a boil in heavy-bottomed soup pot.
2. While waiting for the water to boil, rinse and pick over the
split peas.
3. Add the remaining ingredients and bring back to a boil and
reduce to a simmer. *Note:* Pea soup has to be stirred more often than other soups, since the peas tend to stay at the bottom
of the pot. Allow to simmer about 2 hours. The length of time
it cooks depends on how dry the split peas are.
4. When the split peas are totally dissolved, remove onion, celery,
garlic, and bay leaf to a strainer and taste to correct seasoning.

Serves 10

31 CAL. • 2 G PROTEIN • 5.5 G CARBOHYDRATE • ½ G FAT • 38 MG CHOLESTEROL

Low-Fat Garlic Croutons

Note: Garlic-flavored croutons taste great floating in the soup. I
add a tablespoonful to every bowl served, or you can serve them
separately in their own bowl.

1. Toast several slices of bread and allow to dry out a bit.
2. Rub a peeled clove of garlic over the toast. You may need a
few cloves of garlic.
3. Slice toast into ½-inch-wide strips. Turn toast strips around
and cut across the strips, making pieces ½ inch square, and
serve.

Chicken and Chickpea Soup Flavored with Dill

Although I find all soups satisfying, this is one of those hearty soups that satisfies the spirit as well as the body. The chicken and the chickpeas are very high in protein as well as satisfaction. And, like all soups, the flavor improves in a day or two.

1 tbsp. oil or butter
1 peeled medium onion, finely chopped
2 stalks of celery with leaves, washed and finely chopped
2 large carrots, peeled and finely chopped
2 tbsp. flour
½ tsp. ground sage
2 bay leaves
½ c. white wine
3 c. chicken stock
2 c. water (or all water)
1 c. (or more) raw chicken cut into strips, with no fat,
skin, or bones
1 tsp. Worcestershire sauce
1 20-oz. can chickpeas
¼–½ c. finely minced fresh dill
salt and pepper to taste

1. Heat a heavy-bottomed stockpot and add oil, onion, celery, and carrots. Sauté for a few moments, cover pot, reduce flame, and *sweat* the veggies for about 15 to 20 minutes. They should be softened.
2. Add flour, sage, bay leaves, and white wine and stir. Allow to simmer for about 10 minutes, uncovered.
3. Add stock and water to pot; add Worcestershire sauce; add chicken. Allow to simmer 10 minutes.
4. Add the contents of can of chickpeas to a food processor or a blender and puree.
5. Add puree to the pot and bring back to a simmer.
6. Add salt and pepper to taste.
7. Add fresh dill and simmer for a few moments more.

Note: If you would like a thinner and more chunky soup, don't puree the chickpeas or puree only half the chickpeas.

Serves 4

320 CAL. • 23 G PROTEIN • 42 G CARBOHYDRATE • 5 G FAT • 38 MG CHOLESTEROL

Multi-Bean Soup with Winter Vegetables

With winter veggies and green leafy veggies, this is a high-protein balanced meal, and delicious. Remember, it takes the same amount of work to double or triple the recipe; it stores well in the fridge and freezes well and improves with age. When reheating the next day, you might want to add some leftover (or fresh) greens, such as spinach, chard, chicory, or any kind of lettuce. It adds a fresh flavor to the soup as well as nutrients and fiber.

11 c. cold water or stock
½ c. red kidney beans
½ c. navy beans
½ c. great northern beans
½ c. pinto beans
½ c. dried lima beans

Note: You can substitute almost any dry beans for any of these.

½ c. washed pearl barley
2 bay leaves
1 bouquet garni
1 large onion with root end cut off
2 celery stalks with leaves
1 garlic clove, unpeeled
several sprigs of parsley
5–6 peeled carrots, cut into ½-in. rounds
3–4 peeled red potatoes, cut to about ½-in. cubes
3 turnips, peeled and cut into ½-in. cubes
½ c. canned lentils

½ oz. rinsed dried mushrooms or ¼ lb. fresh sauteed mushrooms
1 tbsp. salt
2 tsp. freshly ground black pepper

1. Rinse and pick over beans.
2. Place all the dried beans (not the lentils) in a large saucepan and cover with cold water. Bring to a boil, reduce to a simmer, and cook for a minute.
3. Drain beans, rinse, and repeat step 2.
4. Place all the beans and barley in a large, heavy-bottomed stockpot. Add the 11 cups cold water or stock, bring to a boil, and reduce to a simmer.
5. Tie the bouquet garni, onion, celery, garlic, and bay leaves in a piece of rinsed cheesecloth and add to the pot.
6. Allow to simmer for about an hour and a half.
7. Add carrots, turnip, and potatoes to pot, cook for about 10 minutes.
8. Add lentils and mushrooms and cook another 10 minutes.
9. Add salt and pepper and parsley.
10. Remove and squeeze the juices out of the cheesecloth package.
11. Taste and adjust seasonings.

Serves 10

240 CAL. • 11 G PROTEIN • 49 G CARBOHYDRATE • UNDER 1 G FAT • 0 CHOLESTEROL

Hummus

This pâté is made up of chickpeas. It's flavored with lemon, garlic, parsley, and other good stuff. Being a type of bean, chickpeas are loaded with protein. Normally this is eaten on a piece of flat bread known as pita. If pita won't go down properly right after surgery, try crackers. Anything crunchy is easier to digest.

1 15-oz. can chickpeas
2–3 cloves finely minced garlic

2 tsp. salt
½ c. tahini
strained juice of 2 lemons
⅓ c. very finely minced parsley
¼ c. minced scallions or chives
About 10–15 turns of a pepper mill
The washed and dried leaves of a head of romaine lettuce

1. Drain chickpeas and place in the bowl of a food processor and pulse several times. It should be mildly grainy.
2. Add the remaining ingredients, except lettuce, to the chickpeas and process. (Careful: If overprocessed it will become too pasty and heavy.)
3. Taste for seasoning. You may prefer more or possibly less garlic and/or lemon.
4. Mound up on a plate or platter and surround with the lettuce leaves or place the leaves on a separate plate. If the leaves are too large cut them in half.

10 servings (as snack or appetizer)

110 CAL. • 5 G PROTEIN • 12 G CARBOHYDRATE • 6 G FAT • 0 CHOLESTEROL

Lentil Menagere

With a little curiosity you can improve your diet markedly, particularly you folks who have to stay away from fat and hard-to-chew food. Well-cooked lentils don't lose texture or flavor. They are usually prepared with contrasting but fatty foods like bacon, but you can use low-fat sausage.

2 c. dry lentils
2 carrots
1 onion
1 turnip
1 celery stalk
1 garlic clove
1 shallot

3 tbsp. oil (olive, peanut, safflower, etc.)
1 tbsp. flour
1 bouquet garni (*see note*)
freshly ground black pepper
salt
optional: 4 links 4-in. pork sausage

1. Wash the lentils and pick them through.
2. Place them in a large pot with cold water and bring to a boil. Have a strainer or colander ready. When they come to a boil, drain.
3. Mince carrots, onion, turnip, celery, garlic, and shallot.
4. In a large sauté pan, heat the olive oil and add minced veggies. Sauté them until they have a golden look and are soft.
5. Add the lentils, bouquet garni, pepper, and a little salt (you can always add additional salt).
6. Add just enough boiling water to barely cover the lentils, reduce to a simmer, cover, and allow to cook for 1½ hours, stirring occasionally.

Note: Bouquet garni is made of several herbs. Usually bay leaf, thyme, and parsley are tied together or tied within cheesecloth and tossed into the pot to be fished out before serving. If using the dry herbs, just sprinkle some into the pot.

Normally this is served with French-style sausages on the side or cut up and cooked with the lentils. I usually steam and then sauté them until they are quite brown. In this way most of the fat is given up. Place 4 links of 4-inch-long pork sausages in about ½ inch water in a heavy-bottom pan. Cover and bring to a boil; allow to simmer for about 10 minutes. Uncover, continue to simmer until the water evaporates. Don't remove the sausages; brown them in the same pan. Slice thin and toss with the lentils.
Serve with a salad and French whole-grain bread.

Serves 5–6

355 CAL. • 22 G PROTEIN • 48 G CARBOHYDRATE • 8 G FAT • 8 MG CHOLESTEROL

BEEF

Beef is an important staple food for WLS patients with any kind of bypass. It is high in both protein and iron—essential nutrients. However, it also tends to be high in fat, so if you want to reduce the fat in these recipes, use a leaner cut of beef or carefully trim the fat off the cut you're using.

Chili

This chili is not the usual kind made with ground beef. It's basically a stew. It's high in protein, and a large amount can be made and frozen for future use. You don't need the added fat of sour cream or cheese for wonderful chili.

2–3 tbsp. vegetable oil
1½ lb. chuck or round steak, cut into medium-size pieces
½ c. chopped onion
2–3 chopped cloves of garlic
1–1½ tsp. chili powder (how hot do you like it?)
½–1 tsp. cayenne pepper (1 dried chili pepper ground)
1 tsp. salt

1. Heat up a seriously large pot with a heavy bottom, add oil and ¼ of the meat immediately. When browned, remove, set aside, and do the next ¼ of the meat, and so on until the entire amount of meat is browned. *Note:* This technique keeps the meat from steaming.
2. Add the onions to the oil remaining after the meat has been removed. Let them sauté for about 4–5 minutes, then add the garlic and allow to cook another 2 minutes.
3. Return meat to pot, cover with cold water, add remainder of the ingredients. Bring to a boil and immediately reduce to a simmer. Allow to simmer at least 4 hours.
4. If you like beans (more protein), this is the time to add about one 16-oz. can of pinto or red kidney beans.

Serves 5–6

Note: Chili will taste better the next day; you can cook it again just before serving. It also freezes very well, so you can divide this up and place in some freezer containers and store for future use.

447 CAL. • 33 G PROTEIN • LESS THAN 1 G CARBOHYDRATE • 33 G FAT •
123 MG CHOLESTEROL

Pepper Steak

No, this is not steak *au poivre,* but my version of a well-known Chinese dish. In this dish the veggies (green pepper) are not as crisp as normally found in Chinese dishes. It makes a lovely high-protein meal.

1 lb. flank, round, or any firm steak
salt and pepper (freshly ground)
2 tbsp. vegetable oil
1 chopped medium onion
2 cloves minced garlic
½ c. dry sherry (fino)
2 c. chopped green bell peppers
1 c. chicken or beef stock
1 c. drained canned tomatoes
2 tbsp. cornstarch
2 tsp. Chinese dark soy sauce
¼ c. water

1. With steak flat on a cutting board in front of you, cut strips about 1½ inches wide. Then turn each piece on its side and slice strips ⅛ inch thick. (This can best be accomplished by freezing the steak slightly.) Sprinkle with salt and pepper.
2. Heat a wok or large skillet. Add the oil and steak strips, brown on both sides, and add onions and garlic.
3. Add the wine, pouring it on the side of the pan or wok, taking care not to pour it directly over contents.
4. Add the peppers, soy sauce, and stock. Simmer about 10 to 12 minutes, then add tomatoes and simmer another 5 minutes.

5. Stir the cornstarch into ¼ cup water and add while stirring the mixture. Cook until it all thickens.

Note: For milder-flavored peppers, before chopping boil halves in water for 2–4 minutes.

Serves 4

581 CAL. • 31 G PROTEIN • 17 G CARBOHYDRATE • 39 G FAT • 14.5 MG CHOLESTEROL

Beef Bourguignon or Beef Stew in Wine
3 lb. stewing beef cut into 2-in. pieces
2 carrots, sliced thin (slice them the long way)
2–3 tbsp. olive oil for browning meat and veggies
large onion, sliced thin
2–3 tbsp. flour
3 c. full-bodied red wine
2–3 c. beef stock, canned beef bouillon, or water
1 tbsp. tomato paste (if you don't have tomato paste, use a good shot of catsup)
2–3 cloves garlic, smashed and peeled
1–2 bay leaves
½ tsp. dried thyme, or a few sprigs of fresh
1½ tsp. salt
Freshly ground black pepper
¼ lb. fresh mushrooms, cut in half (if large, cut into quarters)
2 tbsp. butter (olive oil if you prefer) for sautéing mushrooms

1. Preheat oven to 500 degrees F.
2. Set a small saucepan with the stock on a burner at low to medium heat.
3. While the stock is warming, heat a heavy-bottomed Dutch oven or casserole on the top of the stove.
4. Dry the cut-up pieces of meat with paper towels (moisture will not allow them to brown).
5. When the pot is quite hot, add oil and some of the meat at once. Don't overcrowd; toss the meat about, turning often un-

til it is browned all over. Keep repeating with remaining meat until it is all browned. Set aside the browned meat.

6. Brown the carrots and onions the same way. Truly get them brown (not black); the caramelization (that's what the brown is) adds a great flavor. Set aside.

7. Wipe out the pot you were using for browning and add the meat, tossing it with the 2 tablespoons of flour. Place in the oven for about 5 to 6 minutes. Remove pot from oven, and toss the meat again. Replace the pot in the oven, again for about 5 to 6 minutes. While pot is in the oven, uncork the wine.

8. Remove pot from oven and place on stove. Lower oven temperature to 300 degrees. Over moderate heat, add the boiling stock and the wine. Add salt, pepper, thyme, bay leaf, tomato paste, and garlic. Liquid should barely cover the meat. If not, add a bit more stock or water.

9. As it approaches a boil, remove from heat, cover, and place the pot in the oven. After about 5 minutes, check the stew. It should be just below a simmer—every so often you should see a bubble or two. If it is boiling or simmering, lower the oven about 25 degrees at a time, wait 5 minutes, and check again. It will take about 3½ to 4 hours. Set timer for 3½ hours. At that time test the meat for tenderness; reset timer and keep checking. It should be fork tender.

10. While the meat is in the oven, sauté the mushrooms. Set aside.

11. When done, place the stew in a serving dish with the mushrooms on top. Serve with boiled potatoes or noodles and a fresh salad. A full-bodied red wine goes well with it.

Serves 10 (make this one for a crowd or freeze for future use)

455 CAL. • 44 G PROTEIN • 7.2 G CARBOHYDRATE • 22 G FAT • 288 MG CHOLESTEROL

CHICKEN

Chicken breasts are a good source of animal protein with little fat, and they are lower in cholesterol than most other meats. Chicken can be a problem for WLS patients, however, because the white meat of chicken is so dry and hard to swallow. Years ago I discovered what the Chinese call "Velvet Chicken." Indeed it is as smooth as velvet. The Chinese use it as a partially cooked addition to stir-fried vegetables. You can make this dish to serve on its own, or a few months after surgery make one of the many Chinese stir-fries with veggies.

Velvet Chicken

    1 lb. boneless skinless chicken breast

For velvet coating:

    ½ tsp. salt
    1 tbsp. dry sherry
    1 large egg white
    1 tbsp. cornstarch
    1 tbsp. oil

You may cut the chicken breast in any manner you choose: slices, shreds, dice, or cubes. Shreds may be the best to eat shortly after surgery. *Note:* If frozen (firm but not hard), it is much easier to slice. Wrap in aluminum foil and place in freezer for 2 hours.

For shreds: Slice meat crosswise into about ⅛-inch slices. Stack a few of these slices, then cut along length into shreds. If long, cut in half. They should be about ⅛ by ⅛ by 1½ inches long.

Coating
    1. Place shreds in a bowl.
    2. Add the salt, sherry, and stir.
    3. Beat the egg white until the gel is broken down. Don't beat into a froth; if you do, the coating will puff up and disappear in the cooking.
    4. Add egg whites to the chicken, sprinkle in the cornstarch, and mix well.
    5. Add the tablespoon of oil and stir until quite smooth.

6. Allow the chicken to marinate in the refrigerator for at least 30 minutes; in this way the coating adheres to the meat. (It can also be left overnight in the fridge.)

Velveting

1. Have a strainer or colander ready in your sink. Bring a quart of water to a boil and add a tablespoon of oil to the boiling water.
2. Reduce to a gentle simmer.
3. Scatter in the chicken and separate by stirring. Keep stirring until the coating turns white. Immediately pour through a strainer and cool with cold water to stop the cooking.

Notes about velveting: The oil in the coating prevents lumping up and allows the coating to be lustrous. It also gets rid of the mealiness of cornstarch. The chicken after velveting is not quite fully cooked. If it is not to be stir-fried later, allow it to cook in the water for another minute, but no more than that.

Serves 4

239 CAL. • 36 G PROTEIN • 2.5 G CARBOHYDRATE • 7.5 G FAT • 96 MG CHOLESTEROL

Sautéed Supremes

Most people think of sautéing as frying. Not so. Frying uses oil to some depth, whereas sautéing just coats the pan slightly.

1 boned chicken breast, cut in two (2 supremes)
Flour for dredging
Salt and pepper to taste
2 tsp. olive oil
½ c. dry white wine
½ c. chicken stock (canned is okay)

1. Separate two halves of chicken breast, trimming away fat and membrane.
2. Place on a firm surface between two pieces of plastic wrap and pound to flatten to about ⅜ inch thick. Try for uniform thickness.
3. Heat a heavy pan or skillet until quite hot.

4. While pan is heating, sprinkle meat with flour, salt, and freshly ground pepper. Spread flour mixture with your fingertips and press against the meat. Do the same to the other side. The flour is important: It keeps the moist meat away from the hot pan, which tends to toughen meat.

5. Add olive oil to pan and immediately place meat in pan. After about 1½ to 2 minutes, or when edges become opaque and white, turn and sauté the other side for about 1½ to 2 minutes. Remember, "hot pan cool oil," and nothing will stick.

6. Remove from pan and place on warm dinner plate or on greens that have been placed on warm dinner plate.

7. Having left the heat on, add wine (keep your head back—wine may splatter and flame up), stir to loosen and dissolve any particles that may have stuck to the pan. Add the stock and reduce the liquid in the pan by more than half, enough so that you have about 2 tablespoons per portion. Pour over supremes and serve.

Serves 2

Variation 1: At the end of the reduction, add the juice of half a lemon.

Variation 2: Use white wine alone.

Variation 3: Use white wine and lemon juice.

Variation 4: Substitute Madeira for the white wine in any of the above. (Caution: Madeira will really flame up; the alcohol content is higher.)

Variation 5: At the end of the sauté, add some chopped shallots or mushrooms (or both), sauté for a few moments with the supremes, and further cook them when you do the reduction.

Variation 6: Use stock alone. Instead of greens, use thick wedge-shaped slices of zucchini and yellow summer squash (steam them a little longer, 3 to 4 minutes, along with unflattened supremes). Place supremes and squash on a serving platter.

DON'T BE AFRAID TO MAKE YOUR OWN VARIATIONS— IT'S FUN.

210 CAL. • 29 G PROTEIN • 1.1 G CARBOHYDRATE • 5 G FAT • 73 MG CHOLESTEROL

CHICKEN SALADS WITH A DIFFERENCE

Orange Mayonnaise
(for blender or food processor)

zest of 1 orange (that is the orange part of the peel only)
juice of ½ orange, or 2 tbsp. frozen concentrate
⅓ c. commercial low-fat mayonnaise.
Whip in the orange juice and zest.

3 servings

116 CAL. • ½ G PROTEIN • 15 G CARBOHYDRATE • 7 G FAT • 9 MG CHOLESTEROL

Dill Mayonnaise
Follow recipe for orange mayonnaise, omitting zest and orange juice. Replace with 1 cup loosely packed fresh dill leaves, chopped fine, with large stems removed.

Serves 3

88 CAL. • 0.3 G PROTEIN • 6 G CARBOHYDRATE • 7 G FAT • 9 MG CHOLESTEROL

Chicken Salad

1½ c. prepared sliced velvet chicken
1 large navel orange, peeled and sliced into rounds
1 mango, peeled and sliced (optional)
½ large sweet onion such as Spanish or Vidalia, sliced into rounds
several leaves of red leaf or romaine lettuce, washed and dried

Alternate slices of orange and onion over lettuce leaves; next row, alternate slices of mango and chicken. Serve mayo in a separate bowl in center of platter or pipe it on decoratively, or, while assembling salad, dip half of each piece into mayo.

Serves 2

327 CAL. • 34 G PROTEIN • 33 G CARBOHYDRATE • 7 G FAT • 92 MG CHOLESTEROL

Chicken Salad 2

1½ c. sliced velvet chicken
½ c. chopped celery
3 tbsp. chopped sweet onion
2 tbsp. dill mayonnaise
1 tbsp. minced scallion, including green portion, for garnish

Combine all the ingredients except the scallion. Gently toss in a large bowl and then assemble on a serving platter. Garnish with minced scallion.

Serves 2

212 CAL. • 33 G PROTEIN • 4 G CARBOHYDRATE • 6 G FAT • 92 MG CHOLESTEROL

Coq au Vin Blanc

This dish is quite different from classic Coq au Vin. It is lighter and has many vegetables cooked with it. I find it a great summer treat.

One 3–3½-lb. chicken, cut into serving-size pieces
2–3 tbsp. vegetable oil
1 celery stalk along with some leaves, chopped very thin
1 large onion, sliced into thin rounds
1 clove of garlic, peeled and smashed
3 c. dry white wine
2–3 carrots, depending on size, scraped and cut into 1-in. rounds
1 zucchini, peeled if not organically grown and cut into 1-in. pieces
1 summer squash, peeled if not organically grown and cut into 1-in. pieces
salt and freshly ground pepper
1 bay leaf
2 sprigs of fresh tarragon or ¼ tsp. dried
2–3 sprigs fresh thyme or ¼ tsp. dried

2 large sprigs parsley, chopped very fine
2 tbsp. cornstarch stirred into 3 tbsp. cold water

1. In a large casserole, add oil and heat on a medium-high flame. Season dried chicken pieces with salt and pepper. Sauté until nicely browned and remove from casserole.
2. Sauté onions and celery.
3. Add garlic and sauté another minute or two.
4. Return chicken pieces to the pot, except for breast (white meat).
5. Add wine and ½ tablespoon salt, bring to a boil, and reduce heat to a simmer. Add bay leaf, tarragon, thyme, and parsley.
6. After about 25 minutes add breast pieces, summer squash, carrots, and zucchini. Cook another ten minutes. (White meat tends to dry out when overcooked; dark meat gets more tender with long cooking.)
7. Remove veggies and chicken pieces. Discard bay leaf, raise heat, and reduce liquid to about 2½ cups. Thicken by whisking cornstarch into sauce, and return chicken and veggies to casserole. To increase protein content, at the end of cooking add a can of drained chickpeas and/or frozen young sweet peas, if desired.

Serves 6

335 CAL. • 23 G PROTEIN • 15 G CARBOHYDRATE • 12 G FAT • 65 MG CHOLESTEROL

FISH

Oven-Steamed Fish
If steamed fish seems like a lot of work, here is a simple way of achieving a delightful steamed fish. The French use sealed parchment paper, but we have aluminum foil.

1½ lb. filleted thick white fish, such as cod or sea bass
2 to 3 scallions cut into 2–3-in. pieces
2–3 tbsp. white wine
1–2 tsp. soy sauce

If you happen to find some fresh mushrooms or wild mushrooms, by all means slice some in.

A large piece of aluminum foil, either heavy-duty or doubled.

Preheat oven to 400 degrees F.

1. Place fish in center of foil and fold edges up so that liquids will not run out.
2. Pour wine around fish. Sprinkle soy sauce and scallions over fish.
3. Fold foil around fish, leaving room for steam to circulate. Fold the seams twice over, making it watertight.
4. Place foil package on a cookie sheet or similar tray and place in oven. Steam, allowing 10 minutes per inch of thickness of fish.
5. Remove from oven. Open foil packet carefully—it is full of hot steam. Transfer to platter.

Serves 4–5

173 CAL. • 35 G PROTEIN • 1.7 G CARBOHYDRATE • 1.5 G FAT • 80 MG CHOLESTEROL

Salmon Croquettes

There is almost no fat in this dish. The salmon, along with the egg white, gives us an excellent protein that's easy to digest.

1 can (6 oz.) salmon
1–2 c. leftover mashed potatoes
½ small onion
2 egg whites
½ tsp. salt
1 tsp. (or more) fresh ground black pepper (this dish cries out for a lot of pepper, but you be the judge)
1–2 c. bread crumbs
oil for frying

1. Chop onion and sauté until golden.
2. While the onion is sautéing, drain salmon of liquid and reserve. You might need it if the mix is too dry.

3. Add salmon, onions, egg whites, salt, and pepper to mashed potatoes and mix well with a wooden spoon. If mixture seems too moist, add some bread crumbs. If too dry, add some of the reserved salmon liquid.

4. Put a no-stick or a heavy seasoned cast-iron skillet on the heat.

5. Spread bread crumbs on a platter. From the mixture, form patties about ½ inch thick and place them on the bread crumbs, pressing lightly. Turn them with a spatula (or else they will come apart) and press bread crumbs on the other side.

6. Add a few drops of vegetable oil to the hot skillet and immediately place each croquette in the hot skillet. Reduce heat to low. Cook for about 5 to 7 minutes per side. They should be nicely browned on both sides.

Serves 4

Note: Croquettes can also be made with tuna or minced cooked chicken.

328 CAL. • 17 G PROTEIN • 45 G CARBOHYDRATE • 8 G FAT • 23 MG CHOLESTEROL

Fish Stew or Soup

This is a cross between a soup and a stew. You can use almost any fish or combination of shrimp and fish or clams and fish. If you can't get your fishmonger to give or sell you some fish heads or bones, you can still make a lovely fish stock using parts of the fish you purchase that will normally go to waste. With the addition of clam juice I find it wonderful.

1½ lb. salmon steak or any other rich-tasting fish
4 c. cold water (approx.)
1 celery stalk and some celery leaves
1 medium carrot
1 bay leaf
½ c. white wine
1 medium onion with root end cut off

1 medium potato
1 tsp. salt
1 c. no-fat or low-fat milk

1. Trim away skin and bone and any other part of the fish you won't be eating. Cut fish into 1-inch squares. Reserve the fish pieces.
2. Place skin and bones along with cold water in a 2-quart saucepan and add celery, carrot, bay leaf, onion, and salt.
3. Simmer about an hour or more. Strain through a strainer, making sure to squeeze out as much liquid as possible from the veggies and fish.
4. Taste stock. If not rich enough, add the clam juice.
5. Peel and cut potato into ½-inch cubes.
6. Place potato in the strained stock and cook for about 5 minutes.
7. Add milk and bring back to a simmer.
8. Add reserved fish pieces and simmer about 5 minutes.
9. If desired, at this time add some peeled shrimp and cook about 1 to 2 minutes, depending on size of shrimp or until shrimp turn pink.
10. Taste and adjust with salt and white pepper.

Serves 4–5

310 CAL. • 34 G PROTEIN • 16 G CARBOHYDRATE • 10 G FAT • 80 MG CHOLESTEROL

VEGGIES

Stir-Fried Spinach

Spinach is high in iron, which many post-ops need more of. Once you've tasted spinach done in this manner, you'll never eat it cooked any other way. If the spinach is really young with its typical red roots, leave the roots on; they are very tasty.

About 1 lb. or so of young spinach
1 or 2 garlic cloves
2 tbsp. oil to stir-fry

1 tsp. sugar
1 tsp. salt
2 tsp. sesame oil

1. Place the spinach in a large tub or sink filled with water.
2. Tear off the root ends of the spinach and run water into them (the closed end above the root holds most of the sand).
3. Allow the spinach to sit in the water while you prepare everything else (about 5 to 10 minutes). The sand will be found at the bottom of the sink.
4. Fill a large pot with cold water and bring it to a boil.
5. Collect the spinach into a large colander or strainer and thoroughly rinse under running water.
6. Drain the spinach as best you can and place in the boiling water. Return the colander to the sink.
7. When the water returns to a boil, empty contents of the pot into the colander and run cold water over the spinach immediately to stop the cooking.
8. Once cooled, drain and squeeze out as much water as you can with your hands. At this point you may put the spinach aside to prepare at a later time.

To stir-fry:

1. Peel and smash garlic.
2. Get the wok very hot (but not smoking).
3. Add the 2 tablespoons of oil.
4. Add the garlic, stirring it around and pressing it to extract the juices (you are flavoring the oil). After about 30 seconds of this, discard the garlic.
5. Place the spinach in the hot wok and immediately begin stirring and tossing.
6. Add the sugar and salt, stir for another 30 seconds or so.
7. Turn heat off, add sesame oil, and give one final stir or two.

Serves 2

216 CAL. • 7 G PROTEIN • 11 G CARBOHYDRATE • 18 G FAT • 0 CHOLESTEROL

Steamed Greens

1 small head chicory or escarole or any green leafy vegetable
you prefer, leaves separated, washed, and dried
1 or 2 cloves garlic, peeled and slightly crushed
⅓–½ c. chicken stock or water
2 tbsp. vegetable oil (olive oil is best for flavor)

1. In a large saucepan or wok, heat the oil, add the garlic, and
press against the pan with your spatula or wooden spoon to extract the flavor and oils of the garlic. When garlic starts turning
brown, remove from the pan and discard.
2. Add the greens, tossing and stirring, and watch them turn a
bright green. After about a minute, when they seem to be
bright green all over, add the water or stock.
3. Bring to a boil, cover, and steam for 3 to 4 minutes. Remove
and drain, arrange on one side of warm dinner plate. Serve
with a chicken cutlet, simple vegetable, and potatoes or rice.

Serves 2

171 CAL. • 4 G PROTEIN • 9 G CARBOHYDRATE • 14 G FAT • 0 CHOLESTEROL

INDEX

About the Authors

LOUIS FLANCBAUM, M.D. (pronounced *flans-baum*), is a general surgeon and nationally recognized authority in bariatric surgery. He is the Chief of the Division of Bariatric Surgery at St. Luke's–Roosevelt Hospital Center and associate professor of clinical surgery at the College of Physicians and Surgeons of Columbia University. Dr. Flancbaum is a graduate of the State University of New York—Downstate Medical Center and completed his surgical training at the University of Illinois Medical Center in Chicago and the Maryland Institute for Emergency Medical Services Systems in Baltimore. He has held faculty positions at the University of Medicine and Dentistry of New Jersey–Robert Wood Johnson Medical School, Rutgers University, and the Ohio State University College of Medicine. He is board-certified in General Surgery, Surgical Critical Care, and Nutrition Support. Dr. Flancbaum is a Fellow of the American College of Surgeons (FACS), the American College of Critical Care Medicine (FCCM), and the American College of Chest Physicians (FCCP) and has been elected to membership in over 25 professional societies, including the American Society for Bariatric Surgery, American Society of Clinical Nutrition, American Institute of Nutrition, Society for Surgery of the Alimentary Tract, International Federation for the Surgery of Obesity, and the Society of American Gastrointestinal Endoscopic Surgeons. Dr. Flancbaum has made numerous national and international presentations and has published over 100 articles and book chapters in scientific journals. Dr. Flancbaum lives in Teaneck, New Jersey with his wife Debby. Between them, they have five children; Rachel, Jessica, Meir, Shira and Tova.

Erica Manfred is a freelance writer and medical journalist whose articles on a variety of medical and psychological topics have appeared in *Cosmopolitan; Ladies Home Journal; McCalls; Parenting; Food and Fitness Advisor; Bottom Line/Personal; New Age Journal; Mothers Today; Dr. Joyce Brothers Emotional Health Newsletter;* Healthgate.com; Onebody.com. She had gastric bypass surgery in January of 1998, which substantially improved both her health and quality of life. She lives in Catskill, New York.

Deborah Biskin Flancbaum, M.S., is an educator and freelance writer who contributes to *Lifestyles, Modern Bride,* and *Olam* magazines and Generationj.com. Ms. Flancbaum writes a column featured in the *Jewish Press* entitled, "Dessert with Debby." Ms. Flancbaum edited Dr. Flancbaum's first book, *And You Shall Live by Them; Contemporary Approaches to Jewish Medical Ethics,* and profiled him for *Lifestyles* magazine. She and Dr. Flancbaum are currently collaborating on a book about the meaning of the Jewish holidays. She lives with her husband, Louis Flancbaum, in Teaneck, New Jersey. Between them, the Flancbaums have five incredible children; Rachel Reich, Jessica Levine, Meir, Shira & Tova Flancbaum.